EASY BREAD MAKING

FOR SPECIAL DIETS

Revised Edition

Use your bread machine,
food processor, mixer, or tortilla maker
to make the bread YOU need
quickly and easily

Nicolette M. Dumke

EASY BREADMAKING FOR SPECIAL DIETS, REVISED EDITION: USE YOUR BREAD MACHINE, FOOD PROCESSOR, MIXER, OR TORTILLA MAKER TO MAKE THE BREAD YOU NEED QUICKLY AND EASILY

Published by
Adapt Books
Allergy Adapt, Inc.
1877 Polk Avenue
Louisville, Colorado 80027
303-666-8253

©2007 by Nicolette M. Dumke
Printed in the United States of America
Cover design by Ed Nies, Mel Typesetting,
1523 S. Pearl St., Suite B, Denver, Colorado 80210, 303-777-5571

Publisher's Cataloging in Publication Data

Dumke, Nicolette M.
    Easy Breadmaking for Special Diets: use your bread machine, food processor, tortilla maker, or mixer to make the bread YOU need quickly and easily / Nicolette M. Dumke.
232 p. 24.6 cm.
Includes bibliographical references and index.
LCCN: 2006907350
ISBN-13: 978-1-887624-11-4
ISBN-10: 1-887624 -11-2
1. Bread.   2. Diet therapy.   I. Title
TX769.D86 1996   641.8'15
                                                     QBI95-20288

Dedication

To my husband Mark,
for his encouragement and support
of all of my efforts,

To my son Joel,
for his optimism and positive attitude,

To my son John,
my best helper with this book, who with his
adventuresome spirit tasted every loaf,

And to my many other tasters:
my mother, Mary Jiannetti,
my sister, Gina Jiannetti,
and numerous friends.

Disclaimer

The information contained in this book is merely intended to communicate food preparation material and information about possible treatment options which are helpful and educational to the reader. It is not intended to replace medical diagnosis or treatment, but rather to provide information and recipes which may be helpful in implementing a diet prescribed by your doctor. Please consult your physician for medical advice before embarking on any treatment or changing your diet.

The author and publisher declare that to the best of their knowledge all material in this book is accurate; however, although unknown to the author and publisher, some recipes may contain ingredients which may be harmful to some people.

There are no warranties which extend beyond the educational nature of this book, either expressed or implied, including, but not limited to, the implied warranties of merchantability, fitness for a particular purpose, or non-infringement. Therefore, the author and publisher shall have neither liability nor responsibility to any person with respect to any loss or damage alleged to be caused, directly or indirectly, by the information contained in this book.

If you do not wish to be bound by the above, you may return this book to the publisher for a full refund.

Table of Contents

Foreword

Like the indescribable aroma of fresh baked bread, wafting from the kitchens of our childhoods, comes this wonderful book all about bread.

Easy Breadmaking for Special Diets considers making dozens of different kinds of bread from a wide variety of flours, some of whose names you may have never even heard. It deals with making bread by many techniques, from "by hand" to using the most sophisticated equipment and ovens available. It analyzes the nutritional values of the recipes for you, and shows you how to fit bread into any health-conscious diet.

It offers hope to the environmentally sensitive person who has become resigned to giving up the comfort of having bread as a basic part of any meal. The author shows you how to make really good bread without yeast, milk, eggs, wheat, or salt — all those things you thought were absolutely essential for bread making.

This is a book for people who want to make more bread, for people who want to start making bread, and for people, who because of their allergies, are afraid to make bread. It's all here for you. Enjoy!

Elizabeth Pinar, M.S., R.D.

Medical Nutrition Consultant in private practice
Dietetics Educator – Master Teacher Emeritus,
    Front Range Community College
Author of menu planning software including
    Dinner! for Windows

Bread, the Staff of Life

Bread is the most basic of all foods; it is called the staff of life. Without it, our diets do not seem complete. For 2000 years, people have been asking, "Give us this day our daily bread." The USDA's new food guide pyramid tells us that breads and grains should be the largest part of a health-promoting diet. And yet, those of us on special diets may find it difficult or impossible to purchase commercially made bread that conforms to the diets we must follow for good health.

If you are on a special diet, there is no reason to despair. You can make your own bread quickly and easily. You can take charge of your health and take charge of your life. You will be in control of what you eat and will find that your homemade bread tastes better than any bread you have eaten before. Our homes smell wonderful when we bake. If we want to have bread that will keep us healthy on our special diets, we can make our own.

When you first embark upon a special diet, the challenge of making all of your own bread can seem overwhelming. However, with the many labor-saving devices now available, it does not have to be difficult or take all day like it used to for our grandmothers. Mixers and food processors can do the heavy work of kneading dough, microwave ovens can help it rise in record time, a tortilla maker can press and cook a tortilla all in one operation, or a bread machine can do the whole job of making bread for you from start to finish.

The purpose of this book is to help you achieve good health by following your special diet and to enjoy the simple pleasures of homemade bread while saving you time and effort in the kitchen. The investment you make in good health for yourself and those you love is well worth the effort involved.

Special Diets, Special Recipes

Special diets are used to treat and control a wide variety of medical conditions. Even your family members who consider themselves normal and healthy can benefit from taking control of what goes into their mouths and what goes into their bread. We are what we eat!

Food allergies are commonly treated by avoiding the foods that you are allergic to, such as wheat, milk, eggs, and yeast. Many people cannot handle lactose because they lack the enzyme needed to digest it and so must avoid milk. Individuals with celiac disease must avoid all gluten. Those with hypoglycemia or who are on low-carbohydrate diets for weight control must limit their intake of carbohydrates. People with heart disease or high blood pressure must limit the amount of sodium and/or fat and cholesterol they eat. Diabetics must strictly control the amount of all nutrients and calories they consume, balancing their food intake against their insulin intake or production.

People with intestinal diseases may need either high fiber or low fiber diets. All of us are told that low fat, high fiber diets are good for the prevention of many diseases, such as cancer and heart disease. In this chapter, we will consider some special diets and the recipes in this book that you can use when you are on them.

WHEAT-FREE DIETS

At first glance, a wheat-free diet presents a great challenge to a person baking bread. Wheat is the basic ingredient of almost all commercial bread. Before 1990, those of us with wheat allergies were resigned to eating very dense bread, but with the introduction of spelt to the American market, we once again can make light, fluffy, yet wheat-free breads.

Spelt is a grain that is closely related to wheat. (See page 217 for more information about this). Many individuals who are allergic to wheat can tolerate spelt, but be sure to consult your doctor before trying it. If you can eat spelt, you can have almost any kind of bread you want, and your friends and family may never know it does not contain wheat.

Spelt flour is the basis for many of the wheat-free breads in this book. For those who "rotate" their grains as part of an allergy diet, this book contains recipes for breads made with single grains besides spelt, such as barley, rye, oats, kamut, and rice, and the non-grains, buckwheat, amaranth, and quinoa. (See pages 76, bottom of 78, 79, and bottom of 80 through top of 86). Using these recipes, you can eat bread made with a different grain or non-grain on each day of your rotation diet. If you must also rotate or avoid yeast, refer to pages 124 to the top of 128 for yeast-free, single grain bread recipes.

Over half of the recipes in this book are wheat-free. If you are on a wheat-free diet, avoid those recipes that contain bread flour, all purpose flour, whole wheat flour, whole wheat bread flour, gluten flour, or wheat germ. Also, see the index of wheat-free recipes beginning on page 214.

GLUTEN-FREE DIETS

People with celiac disease (gluten sensitive enteropathy) must avoid all gluten in their diets. Although independent testing laboratories, such as the Rodale Institute, find grains such as millet, milo, and teff and the non-grains amaranth, quinoa, and buckwheat to be essentially gluten-free, at the time of this writing the Celiac Sprue Association has not yet tested these flours and recommends eating breads made from only rice, potato, tapioca, arrowroot, corn, and legume flours. For gluten-free recipes acceptable to the Celiac Sprue Association, refer to the listing of rice recipes on page 215.

MILK- AND LACTOSE-FREE DIETS

It may be necessary to avoid milk products in the diet for several reasons. Some individuals lack the enzyme lactase that breaks lactose (milk sugar) down into glucose and galactose. When the undigested lactose enters the intestine, it causes cramping, gas, and diarrhea. Often lactase-deficient people can tolerate small amounts of milk products, such as the amounts usually found in commercial breads, or can use lactase-treated milk in their diets.

Others must avoid milk in their diets because of allergy to the protein components of milk. These people must usually strictly avoid all milk in their foods. If tolerated, soy or rice milk may be used as a milk substitute in cooking, but it usually works just as well to substitute water. All of the recipes in this book are milk- and lactose-free and are suitable for those on milk- and lactose-free diets. Milk or cheese is an optional ingredient in the recipes for "White Bread," page 60, "Calzones," pages 157 and 159, "Mexican Strata," page 158, and "Pizza," pages 154 to 156, but can easily be omitted without affecting the quality.

EGG-FREE DIETS

Your doctor may recommend an egg-free diet for a variety of reasons. The most common reason today is to control cholesterol levels for the prevention or treatment of heart disease. Most of the recipes in this book are egg-free. A few of the gluten-free recipes require eggs to give structure to the bread, but if you are avoiding eggs to control your cholesterol, a cholesterol-free egg substitute may be used in place of the eggs in these recipes, and is given as an alternative ingredient.

Those who must avoid eggs in their diet because of food allergies should also avoid egg substitutes because they contain egg white, which for most people is the most allergenic part of the egg. Only the cholesterol-rich yolk has been removed in commercial egg substitutes. Egg substitutes may also contain milk or milk derivatives, corn derivatives, or even wheat gluten, all of which can be very allergenic. If you are allergic to both gluten-containing grains and eggs, you may have to settle for dense bread, but such bread is still much better than no bread at all.

SUGAR-FREE DIETS

At our house we have a saying, "Sugar isn't good for anybody." In our experience, we have found that eliminating sugar from our diets is the best way to control our weight without feeling hungry, counting calories, limiting portion sizes, or making any other changes. On a sugar-free diet, wide swings in blood sugar levels, which can lead to excessive hunger and overeating, are uncommon. Eating a large amount of sugar may also predispose to the development of dental cavities, candidiasis, heart disease (by raising the level of blood fats), adult onset diabetes (by "wearing out" the pancreas), and a number of other diseases.

Sugar can be replaced in your diet with fruit and fruit sweeteners. Once your taste buds have become used to a sugar-free diet, you will find that treats made with fruit sweeteners are just as delicious and satisfying as those made with sugar. All of the recipes in this book are sugar-free except for the optional sweet roll and doughnut glazes. Honey may be substituted for liquid fruit sweeteners if it is easier for you to find in your store. It is given as an optional alternative ingredient to fruit sweeteners in some of the sweet bread and roll recipes for those whose taste buds may desire a little more intensely sweet taste than the fruit sweeteners contribute. Molasses is used in the pumpernickel bread, brown bread, and gingerbread recipes.

YEAST-FREE AND LOW YEAST DIETS

Yeast is a common food allergen, and must be avoided by many people with food allergies or who have candidiasis. However, it is possible to make very enjoyable yeast-free breads. There are several bread machines on the market that have a cake or quick bread cycle that can make yeast-free breads. Making yeast-free breads by hand is also very easy. For yeast-free bread and tortilla recipes, see pages 54 to 55 and pages 123 to 150. Also be sure to read "All About Tortillas" and "All About Quick Breads" on pages 16 to 19.

HEART HEALTHY, LOW FAT, LOW CHOLESTEROL DIETS

People on heart healthy diets are usually advised to control the amount of saturated fat and cholesterol they consume. All of the recipes in this book are made with minimal amounts of oil rather than saturated fats such as butter or margarine. Some types of oil, such as canola or olive oil, may be considered better for the prevention or treatment of heart disease than other kinds of oils. Ask your doctor or nutritionist what type of oil you should use.

As mentioned above in the section on egg-free diets, except when necessary to add structure to gluten-free breads, all of the recipes in this book are egg-free. If you are not allergic to eggs or the other ingredients in commercial egg substitutes and wish to make gluten-free breads, you may want to use an egg substitute to avoid the cholesterol in eggs. A few recipes in this book, most of them in the main dish chapters, pages 151 to 173, contain a small amount of cholesterol, but most of the recipes in this book are free of all saturated fat and cholesterol. Refer to the nutritional analyses of specific recipes to see if the saturated fat and cholesterol level in them is low enough to conform to the diet your doctor has given you.

LOW SODIUM DIETS

A low sodium or low salt diet may be recommended for the treatment of high blood pressure, heart disease, or kidney disease. Most of the sodium in our diets comes from salt added to foods. Low sodium bread is a special challenge because salt moderates and controls the growth of the yeast in bread and also contributes to the strength of the gluten structure. Therefore, omitting salt in a type of bread that has a less-than-perfect gluten structure to begin with will cause the bread to fall. A few recipes that contain no added salt are included in this book. (See pages 60, 62, and 66). If you are on a sodium restricted diet and wish to make the other recipes using less salt, the amount of salt in the recipe may be cut in half, which will almost cut the sodium content of the bread in half, without affecting the quality of the bread too much, although the taste will be different. Or consider eliminating the salt from what you put on the bread (butter, nut butter, meat, etc.) rather than from the bread itself.

HIGH FIBER DIETS

High fiber diets are recommended for the treatment of constipation, diverticulosis, irritable bowel syndrome, and hemorrhoids. A high fiber diet may also help stabilize blood sugar levels for diabetics and hypoglycemics by slowing down and stabilizing the rate at which glucose is absorbed from the digestive system. High fiber diets also help control blood cholesterol levels and may help prevent cancer and heart disease.

There are two types of fiber, soluble and insoluble. Insoluble fiber, such as is present in wheat bran and rice bran, passes through the digestive system unchanged and prevents constipation. Soluble fiber, such as is present in apples, barley, and oats, is broken down by the bacteria in the large intestine. It is useful for the prevention of cancer and heart disease.

Grains in general and many of the breads in this book are good sources of fiber. For high fiber bread recipes, refer to pages 45 to 46, 49 to 50, 65 to 68, and "Whole Grain and Extra-Nutrition Breads," pages 73 to 88.

LOW FIBER DIETS

People who have inflammatory bowel disease (IBD) may need to eat low fiber diets to keep from further irritating their intestine. I "discovered" white spelt flour while trying to find low fiber wheat alternatives for a friend who has ulcerative colitis. While insoluble fiber can be a problem for those with IBD, soluble fiber can be a friend. Oatmeal is often recommended as a home remedy for flare-ups because it contains abundant soluble fiber which absorbs water and slows transit time through the intestine. Because I am allergic to grains, I never tried the "oatmeal remedy," but when I had active Crohn's disease before EPD/LDA treatment, I found other soluble fibers, such as psyllium seed, guar gum, and apple pectin, helpful. For more information about EPD/LDA treatment and IBD or irritable bowel syndrome, see *The Ultimate Food Allergy Cookbook and Survival Guide* as described on the last pages of this book.

Many of the basic bread recipes in this book are low enough in fiber for a low fiber diet. Refer to the nutritional analyses of the recipes to get an idea of how much fiber each recipe contains and how likely you are to tolerate it. Much of the fiber in the oatmeal breads, pages 67 to 68, is soluble fiber so oatmeal bread may be tolerated better than the oat bran breads or other whole grain breads which are high in insoluble fiber. Also, in addition to many white spelt bread recipes, there are rice bread recipes that can be made with white rice flour rather than brown rice flour (see pages 52, 55, 72, and 152) and white rye flour recipes (see pages 51, 79, 81, and 126) that may be useful for those on low fiber diets.

DIABETIC DIETS

Diabetics must strictly control their intake of calories and nutrients and balance their food consumption against their insulin intake or their body's production of insulin. This is usually accomplished by using a system of "exchanges" to budget and control their intake of various nutrients. Your doctor or dietician will work out a diet for you which will specify how many and what types of food exchanges to eat at each meal and snack. The serving sizes for the recipes in this book have been geared to the diabetic exchange system. For example, the nutritional analysis for a dense, whole grain bread may say that a large loaf of bread contains 22 servings. Each serving will contain about 80 calories and 15 grams of carbohydrate and be one starch/bread exchange. However, when you make the bread in a bread machine, you may get a loaf which is difficult to cut into 22 slices. A diabetic can cut the loaf into 11 horizontal slices and count each half slice as one starch/bread exchange. A person who is not a diabetic and with no need to count calories may eat a full-sized slice as one serving and get twice as many calories and other nutrients in their serving.

All of the recipes in this book contain a nutritional analysis which specifies how many servings the recipe makes and how many exchanges each serving is. By dividing the loaf of bread (or other recipe) into the number of servings specified, you can easily use these recipes on a diabetic diet.

CARBOHYDRATE CONTROLLED DIETS

Carbohydrate controlled diets are useful for people with hypoglycemia or those who follow a low carbohydrate diet for weight loss. By eating only a moderate amount of carbohydrate (preferably complex carbohydrate) at one time and balancing it with protein, spikes in blood sugar levels, followed by plummeting blood sugar resulting in hunger, can be avoided. For more information about controlling blood sugar levels for weight loss by using a carbohydrate controlled diet, see *Easy Cooking for Special Diets* as described on the last pages of this book.

This book contains a high-protein bread recipe (page 90) which may be useful for a carbohydrate controlled diet. Also, the pita bread and tortilla recipes in this book can be used to make "wraps" or pita sandwiches (put the sandwich fillings into a half-pita) which are lower in carbohydrates than an ordinary sandwich. Both this book and *Easy Cooking for Special Diets* give nutritional analyses for all of the recipes. You can use these numbers to count grams of carbohydrate and control your carbohydrate intake.

LOW CALORIE DIETS

Bread, by nature, is a low fat food containing a moderate number of calories. What can make nutritious, whole grain, high fiber bread a high-calorie snack is putting a lot of butter or bologna on it! When you make your own fresh bread, you may find that it has so much flavor that you do not need to put butter on it to make it enjoyable. All of the breads in this book are sugar-free which may help with weight control more than counting calories. (See "Sugar-Free Diets," page 10). If you do want to count calories, the nutritional analysis given with each recipe in this book will allow you to do so easily.

HOW TO USE THE NUTRITIONAL ANALYSES OF
THE RECIPES IN THIS BOOK

Each recipe in this book is followed by a nutritional analysis.[*] This analysis contains the number of calories, grams of protein, grams of carbohydrate, grams of fat (total and saturated), milligrams of cholesterol, milligrams of sodium, and grams of fiber per serving. If you divide the recipe or cut the loaf of bread into the number of servings specified in the recipe, you can use the "per serving" values given to find out, for instance, how many calories a serving of the bread contains.

For some of the recipes, such as a sweet roll dough recipe, the nutritional analysis is given for the whole recipe. If you use this dough to make another recipe, such as cinnamon rolls, add the whole-recipe values for the dough to the values given in the cinnamon roll recipe for the added ingredients, such as raisins, oil, and sweeteners, and divide by the number of rolls you made to get the nutritional values for each roll.

If a recipe gives a choice between ingredients, the nutritional analysis will be based on the first choice given. If there are significant nutritional differences between two choices, such as between egg substitutes and eggs, a nutritional analysis will be given for both choices. If a recipe includes optional ingredients, the nutritional analysis will be based on

---

[*] Most of the nutritional analyses in this book were calculated from the nutritional values of foods from several sources, including *Foods and Nutrition Encyclopedia* by Audrey H. Ensminger, M. E. Ensminger, James E. Kolande, and John R. K. Robinson, M.D., Pegus Press, 1983, *Perspectives In Nutrition* by Gordon M.Wardlaw, Ph.D., R.D., L.D. and Paul M. Insel, Ph.D., Mosby College Publishing, 1990, and information supplied by the producers of several of the food ingredients. The nutritional analyses of the recipes which are new to the revised edition of this book were calculated using the computer program "The Food Processor for Windows" by ESHA. Every effort has been made to insure that these analyses are as accurate as possible. However, since they are based on values that were measured from a limited number of samples of the foods involved, they are, by their very nature, approximations.

making the recipe without the optional ingredients. If a range is given for the amount of an ingredient to use (for example, if the recipe says to use 1 to 2 cups of an ingredient) the nutritional analysis will be based on the first amount given.

For those who are not counting calories and are not on diabetic diets, the nutritional analyses may be used in a more general, comparative way. For instance, if you want to increase the amount of fiber in your diet, use the nutritional analyses to compare the grams of fiber per serving for two different kinds of bread when deciding which one to make. You can compare the amount of fat or saturated fat in a doughnut made from one of the recipes in this book to that in a commercially made doughnut and see just how much good you are doing yourself or your family by making your own freshly baked doughnuts. Use the nutritional analyses as general guidelines to help make wise choices about what you will eat.

THE BOTTOM LINE – YOUR DIET

What should we do nutritionally to insure good health? According to Dr. Leo Galland, a pioneer in combining conventional medicine with the best insights of alternative medicine, we should eat a nutrient-dense diet for optimal health. This means eating foods that have the greatest number of nutrients for the number of calories you will be consuming. Eat unprocessed or minimally processed foods whenever possible. If you have food allergies, avoid your allergenic foods. If you are overweight or have blood sugar problems, choose your foods to minimize major swings in your blood sugar level which can produce hunger which is out-of-line with what you really need. Ask your doctor for specific information about any special diet you need to follow.

Practically speaking, how do you go about getting a nutrient-dense diet? By making wise decisions about what to eat. Do not choose foods solely by strict counting of calories (but follow your prescribed exchange plan if you are a diabetic) but by thinking about nutrients as well and using common sense. When you want a snack, skip that sugary store-bought pastry made from highly refined flour and fried in hydrogenated fat. Instead choose a piece of fresh fruit, some nuts, or whole grain bread with a little natural nut butter or cheese. Learn to cook and then do it for most meals. The recipes in this book and the other books described on the last pages of this book will help you cook for yourself easily and economically. Plan meals based on nutritious whole foods in advance and grocery shop based on your meal plans. Take charge of your diet and your health. It's the best investment of both time and money that you can make.

All About Tortillas

What is a tortilla? It is a versatile unleavened flatbread which can be eaten alone or can accompany a meal, be made into chips, or become the foundation of a tremendous variety of delicious Mexican main dishes. It is the basic all-purpose ingredient of Mexican cuisine from appetizers to desserts.

The ingredients that make up a tortilla are simple: flour, water, usually a little salt, and sometimes some oil. Since tortillas are unleavened, they can be made with a wide variety of flours, some of which cannot be made into almost any other kind of baked product. This makes tortillas a welcome addition to the diets of people with severe food allergies.

The dough for tortillas is easily mixed by hand, but rolling and cooking them can be a difficult and time-consuming process. Tortillas made from wheat and spelt flours hold together well and can be rolled on a floured board with a rolling pin. The other types of tortillas must be rolled between two pieces of waxed or parchment paper. (This paper is peeled off before cooking them). Mexican cooks use tortilla presses to simplify the rolling process. Rather than using a rolling pin, the ball of dough is placed between pieces of waxed paper and placed in the press near the hinge. Then the handle is pressed down to create a very round tortilla in an instant.

To make tortillas by hand, make the dough and form it into balls 1 to 1½ inches in diameter, or about the size of a small plum. Flatten each ball slightly. If you are making wheat or spelt tortillas, you may roll the balls out on a floured surface to about ⅛ inch thickness. For all other types of tortillas, place the flattened ball of dough between two pieces of wax or parchment paper. Use a rolling pin to roll it out to about 6 or 7 inches in diameter.

Preheat an ungreased skillet or heavy griddle over medium-high heat. If you have used waxed paper to roll the tortilla, carefully peel the paper off of one side. Put the tortilla on the pan with dough side down and cook it for about 30 seconds to one minute; then peel off the second piece of waxed paper from the top of the tortilla. Continue cooking it until it is dry around the edge, one to two minutes more. Turn the tortilla with a spatula and cook the second side for another two to three minutes. Wheat and spelt tortillas will form blisters. Cook tortillas made from wheat and spelt until the blisters begin to brown. Most of the other types of tortillas should not brown; they should be set but not firm when they are finished cooking. Kamut tortillas will often form blisters that brown on the second side of the tortilla cooked; this also occasionally happens with lower gluten tortillas such as barley tortillas.

An electric tortilla maker simplifies the process of making and cooking tortillas tremendously much as much as a bread machine simplifies making yeast bread. To use an electric tortilla maker, first open it, plug it in, and begin preheating it. Mix the tortilla dough as directed in the recipe. Divide the dough into balls about 1 to 1½ inches in diameter, or about the size of a small plum. The dough for tortillas made with all-purpose or unbleached flour should be allowed to "rest" for one-half hour at this point in the process.

When the iron has finished preheating, flatten a ball of dough slightly and place it on the bottom plate of the tortilla maker about halfway between the center and the edge nearest the hinge of the press. Press down the handle in one quick movement. (Wheat, spelt and kamut tortillas can be re-pressed if they are not large enough, but this does not work well with the other types of tortillas. They may blow apart into many pieces if you repress them). After a few tortillas, you will know how much to press to form a tortilla of the desired size without pressing so hard that the edges become lacy. Open the iron immediately after pressing and allow the tortilla to cook until it becomes dry on the bottom side, or for the time directed in your tortilla maker's instruction booklet. Turn it over using a spatula that is safe for non-stick surfaces. Cook the second side until it is also done. As in making hand-cooked tortillas, for most types of tortillas "done" means dry. For wheat and spelt tortillas, cook them until the blisters just begin to brown on both sides.

After cooking your tortillas, remove them from the tortilla maker, griddle, or skillet to a cooling rack and allow them to cool completely. Then stack them and store them in a plastic bag in the refrigerator. Warm tortillas are a wonderful accompaniment to a meal. To reheat them, wrap them in aluminum foil and heat them in a 350° oven for ten to fifteen minutes or microwave them on high for six to seven seconds per tortilla.

Once you have tortillas, you can make them into a myriad of delicious and nutritious main dishes, snacks, and even desserts. Add some excitement to your life and expand the variety of your meals using the tortilla-based recipes on pages 161 to 173.

All About Quick Breads

What is quick bread? Like yeast bread, it is flour, water or other liquid, and usually a little salt and sweetener, but it is leavened by the chemical reaction between baking soda and an acid ingredient rather than by the action of yeast. Because there is no need for yeast to grow and multiply, it is baked immediately after mixing and therefore can be made more quickly than yeast bread.

When baking soda is mixed with an acid ingredient in a liquid environment, carbon dioxide gas is immediately formed. This gas is trapped in the batter or dough and will be baked as little bubbles into the final product. There are many different acid ingredients that you can use. Cream of tartar and unbuffered vitamin C crystals are two dry acid ingredients. Baking powder consists of a dry acid ingredient plus baking soda and some starch (usually cornstarch) to keep the baking soda and acid apart and dry until you are ready to bake. Quick breads can also be made with a wide variety of liquid acid ingredients such as fruit juices, vinegar, or buttermilk.

There are many kinds of non-yeast bread products besides bread: muffins, biscuits, crackers, granola, waffles, pancakes, and cakes are just a few of them. If you need to make these items for use on an allergy diet, refer to *The Ultimate Food Allergy Cookbook and Survival Guide* or *Allergy Cooking with Ease,* described on the last pages of this book.

There are several bread machines on the market that have a quick bread or cake cycle that can make yeast-free bread for you from start to finish. If you understand the process of making quick breads by hand you will find it easier to make quick bread using these machines.

To make non-yeast breads by hand, combine the dry ingredients in a bowl. These usually consist of flour, salt, spices, and dry leavening ingredients, such as baking powder, baking soda, cream of tartar, or vitamin C crystals. (If you must avoid baking powder because of allergy to the starch component, which is usually corn, you can use baking soda in conjunction with an acid ingredient, such as unbuffered vitamin C crystals, cream of tartar, citrus juice, vinegar, buttermilk, or acid fruit juices, or you can use Featherweight™ baking powder, which contains potato starch). Combine the liquid ingredients in a separate bowl or cup. These include water, oil, fruit juice, fruit purees, eggs, liquid acid leavening ingredients, etc.

It is very important to preheat your oven and to oil and flour your baking pans before you mix the liquid and dry ingredients together. The chemical reaction that produces leavening begins immediately upon mixing and may be finished before you get the bread into the oven if there is any delay. When everything is ready, and you do not think the phone is going to ring or you will be otherwise interrupted, quickly stir the liquid ingredients into the dry ingredients. It is more important to be quick than thorough about this; if some lumps or dry spots remain, do not worry. Over mixing is much more likely to cause problems with quick breads than under mixing. Put the batter into the prepared pan and bake, usually at 350°F, for 35 minutes to an hour depending on the type of bread. To test non-yeast breads for doneness, insert a wooden toothpick into the center of the loaf. If it comes out dry, the bread is done. The loaf should also be nicely browned.

As in making quick breads by hand, when you make quick breads in a bread machine, it is important that the batter not be over-mixed. The ideal mixing time for the recipes in this book is three to four minutes. (This may follow a minute or two of slow mixing). If your machine mixes quickly for longer than four minutes, add the oil as directed in the recipe, but delay adding the other liquid ingredients until about two minutes before the end of the mixing time. For example, if it mixes for six minutes, rather than adding the liquids (other than oil) one and one-half to two minutes into the cycle, wait until four minutes after you start the machine.

Quick breads made without eggs or fruit purees can be quite fragile. It is important to cool these breads completely on a rack before slicing them. But if you make a very sturdy bread such as banana bread, go ahead and enjoy it as soon as it comes out of the oven or bread machine.

I store most quick breads in a plastic bag at room temperature or in the freezer. However, some of the fruit-containing breads can be quite moist, so I might keep them in the refrigerator to prevent mold growth if they are not getting eaten quickly. Quick breads do not seem to get stale in the refrigerator as readily as yeast breads do.

For those on yeast-free or low yeast diets, quick breads fill a very important gap in your diet. For everyone, non-yeast breads are quick and easy to make, provide variety in your diet, and the fruit-containing quick breads and cakes are great desserts.

All About Yeast Breads

What is yeast bread? At the most basic level, it is flour, water, and usually a little salt and sweetener. The miracle worker that makes these simple ingredients into one of our most delicious foods is yeast, with the proper application of heat and the development of a good structure (usually gluten) of the bread dough.

Yeast is single celled microorganism and is what makes yeast breads rise and become the light, fluffy, flavorful delights that we expect them to be. The yeast does this by producing carbon dioxide gas which is trapped in the structure of the bread and causes it to expand.

Several factors influence this process. The most important is the temperature at which the yeast grows and multiplies. When yeast breads are made by hand, the dough should be kept at about 85 to 90°F during the rising process, both initially after the dough is made and after the dough is shaped and put in the pan for the second rise before baking.

The proper temperature of the water used to dissolve the yeast varies depending on the method you are using to make the dough. When making bread by hand or using a mixer, the temperature of the water should be about 115°F because the bread will cool as it kneads. When using a bread machine or food processor, the water should be at or slightly above room temperature, about 80°F, because the bread machine or food processor will heat up the dough slightly as it kneads. The other ingredients that are put into the bread should all be at about room temperature.

There are two almost-foolproof ways to create a cozy place for your yeast bread to rise (or "proof") if you are making it by hand, mixer, or food processor. One is to heat your electric oven to 350°F for five minutes, turn it off, and leave the door open until it cools to about 90°F. (A yeast thermometer is an essential tool for checking both the temperature of your rising place and the water used to dissolve the yeast). Then close the door and you will have a warm, draft-free rising place for your bread. Or if you have a gas stove, the pilot light will keep the inside of the oven at the right temperature for bread dough to rise.

The second method of keeping your yeast bread at the right temperature during its rising time is to use a microwave oven with multiple power settings. In a microwave, your yeast bread will rise more quickly and save you time, although initially it will take a little experimentation to determine the right setting to use for each microwave oven. To use your microwave to proof your bread, see pages 24 to 25.

In addition to the proper temperature, other factors influence the growth of yeast. One is the availability of food. Most bread recipes contain some type of sugar (usually fruit sugar in this book) to nourish the yeast, although Italian, French, and sourdough breads do not. (In these types of bread, the yeast is nourished more slowly as the enzymes in the flour break down some of the starch into sugar). Acidity influences the growth of the yeast. Yeast prefers slightly acid conditions, but too much acid, such as is encountered when you try to make the dough very sweet using fruit sweeteners, can inhibit the growth of the yeast. Salt also moderates the growth of yeast. Bread made without salt will rise much faster and higher, and may fall during baking if it over-proofs (rises too much).

The gas made by the yeast must be trapped by the bread dough to cause the dough to rise. In breads made with wheat and spelt and to a lesser degree rye and kamut, the gluten naturally present in the flour is developed during the kneading process into a network of fibers which traps the gas. Kneading causes small molecules of the gluten proteins to form long chains and sheets. This makes the dough feel smooth and elastic, and when you poke your finger into it, it will spring back. The gas made by the yeast is trapped in this gluten structure, and the result is light, fluffy bread.

There are several methods of kneading bread dough to properly develop the gluten structure. The most basic is old fashioned hand kneading. The yeast bread recipes in this book can be made this way if desired; hand kneading is a therapeutic activity if you have the energy for it. If you are interested in making your bread with less effort, you can knead it using a mixer or food processor as described on pages 43 to 53. And of course, a bread machine does all of the kneading automatically, as well as controlling the rising time, maintaining the right temperature, and baking the bread.

If you wish to make gluten-free breads, such as rice, buckwheat, quinoa, or amaranth bread, or breads that contain only a small amount of gluten, such as barley or oat bread, you will have to add something to trap the gas and strengthen the structure of the bread. The most common ingredients to add are guar gum or xanthum gum. Both are soluble fibers that form into chains during kneading. They are not as strong as gluten, so if the dough rises too much, your bread will fall during baking. Other ingredients, such as tapioca flour and eggs, also help to strengthen the structure of gluten-free or low gluten breads. The structure of these breads is best developed by a mixer or bread machine.

All yeast bread making is based on the handmade bread process, so in order to understand making yeast breads in a bread machine, an understanding of the hand process is valuable. Also, if you wish to make the recipes in this book by hand, you can do so by this process. Or, if you wish to make dough in your bread machine and then bake it into a more conventional shape, you can finish the second rising and baking by this process.

To make yeast bread by hand, begin by combining the water and sweetener called for in the recipe in a bowl. Sprinkle the active dry yeast over the surface of the liquid and allow it to stand for ten to fifteen minutes or until it bubbles or "proofs." Stir in the salt, oil, and about half of the flour, and beat it until it is elastic. Stir in as much of the remaining flour as you can, and then turn the dough out onto a floured board to knead it. Knead it by pushing on it with the heels of your hands, folding it over, turning it 90 degrees, and then repeating the process over and over for about ten minutes, gradually adding more flour, until the dough is smooth and elastic. The "feel" of the bread will tell you when enough flour has been added; it will no longer be sticky and will be very resilient. Hand-kneaded bread will absorb a little more flour than called for in most bread machine recipes. Other ingredients, such as nuts and raisins, may be added during this kneading time.

Put the dough in an oiled bowl, and turn it over to oil the other side of the dough. Cover it with plastic wrap or a towel, and allow it to rise in a warm place such as your oven as described above, or microwave until it has doubled in volume. In an oven, this will take 45 to 60 minutes for most kinds of breads. In a microwave (this method is described on pages 24 to 25), it will take about fifteen minutes. If quick-rise yeast is used instead of active dry yeast, the rising time will be about one-third shorter.

Punch the dough down and form it into a loaf, rolls, or whatever shape you desire. Place it into an oiled pan and allow it to rise until doubled again. If your dough is rising in the oven or a warm spot in your kitchen, the second rise will take less time than the first rise. If you are using the microwave method of proofing your dough (described on pages 24 to 25), the second rise will take about fifteen minutes. To tell when gluten-containing dough is ready to bake, poke it gently with your finger. If it does not spring back, it is ready. Gluten-free or non-gluten doughs should be judged visually by looking at their size. It is better to bake them when they are only 1¾ times their original volume than to let them over-proof or they may collapse during baking.

If you are proofing the bread in your oven, take it out when it has risen enough. Preheat the oven to 350°F or 375°F for most loaf breads or 375°F for most rolls. Bake from 15 to 25 minutes for rolls. Light, fluffy, gluten-containing breads will take 45 minutes to an hour to bake. Dense whole grain, low-gluten, or non-gluten breads can take over an hour to bake. The bread is done when it is brown and pulls away from the sides of the pan. To keep the crust from getting soggy, remove the bread from the pan immediately after baking. For light, fluffy, gluten-containing breads, if you tap the bottom of the loaf and it sounds hollow, it is done. The more dense breads may not sound hollow but should be well browned. If sweet breads brown too rapidly during baking, cover them with a piece of foil partway through the baking time.

Most experts recommend letting your bread cool off before you cut it and eat it. However, around our house, it smells so good that some of the little people can't wait that long. I have found that if I use a good bread knife and a gentle sawing motion to cut it, I can cut it immediately without smashing the loaf, although the cut edge may not be as nice as if it had completely cooled before I cut it. You may be able to purchase a good bread knife such as a Henckels in a discount store, as I did, for a fraction of the price that they sell for in cooking catalogues or stores. My knife is probably not "top of the line," but it works very well.

Homemade bread keeps best when stored at room temperature or in the freezer. It gets stale more quickly in the refrigerator. Always let your bread cool completely before storing it. A good, economical way to store bread is in a plastic bag on the kitchen counter. The crust will soften in a plastic bag. Some people use paper or waxed paper bags to store bread if they want the crust to stay crisp. The King Arthur Flour Baker's Catalogue carries perforated polyethylene coated paper bags that are good for storing bread.

An old-fashioned bread box is also a good place to store homemade bread. You do not need to use plastic bags when you store bread in a good bread box. If you want to see how bread keeps in a bread box before buying one, store some rolls in a metal pan with a snug-fitting lid.

In recent years, many bread boxes have become more decorative than functional and may allow the bread to dry out rapidly. The only brand I've found that works well recently is a stainless steel bread box with a frosted glass roll top which is made by WMF. It is sold in Williams Sonoma stores, in their catalogue, and on their website at the time of this writing.

Homemade bread can be a budget stretcher. Some family members who might balk at having soup for dinner think freshly made bread or rolls with soup is a great treat and look forward to soup-and-bread nights. Such meals are much more in line with the USDA's new food guidelines than traditional meals as well. If you are cooking for a special diet and can find commercial bread you can eat, it may cost over $3 for a small loaf, so for special breads, the money you save by making your own can really add up over a period of time.

Homemade yeast breads are one of life's most basic simple pleasures. May this book introduce you to the enjoyment of easily making your own.

Let's Make It Easy: Equipment to Help You

We have many advantages our grandmothers did not have when it comes to making bread. Instead of having to use short-lived compressed yeast, we have very reliable active dry yeast. We can make our bread with appliances we already have, such as our mixers and food processors, and use our microwave ovens to cause it to rise quickly. Or, we can use a bread machine to do everything but measure the ingredients for us. Today bread making is a joy rather than a chore. This chapter will explore some of the appliances that can help you make bread quickly and with minimal effort.

ELECTRIC TORTILLA MAKERS

Making tortillas by hand can make producing homemade yeast bread look easy! Gluten-free tortillas, such as traditional corn tortillas, must be rolled between waxed or parchment paper or pressed with a tortilla press. Then they must be peeled off the paper and cooked on a griddle or skillet one at a time. Although wheat and spelt tortillas are easier to make, they still require considerable effort. An electric tortilla maker greatly simplifies both the rolling and cooking parts of the tortilla-making process.

An electric tortilla maker is a tortilla press with a heating unit in the bottom. After making the dough, you place a small ball of it on the bottom plate, press it to the desired thickness, and then open the press while the tortilla cooks on one side. There is no need to transfer the tortilla at any time. When the bottom of the tortilla is cooked, use a spatula that is safe for non-stick surfaces to turn the tortilla and cook the other side. Because you don't have to transfer the tortilla when you use an electric tortilla maker, people with food allergies can make tortillas using the most delicate, difficult-to-work-with types of flours they might need for their diets using an electric tortilla maker.

MICROWAVE OVENS

As mentioned on page 20, you can use your microwave oven to warm your yeast bread and cause it to rise much more quickly than it normally would. Using a food processor and microwave, you can make homemade bread in just two hours. Your microwave must have an adjustable power setting. Most microwave ovens made now can be set at a low enough power to warm your bread dough without killing the yeast. However, you will have to experiment a little to find the power level and time that works best for your microwave.

To use the microwave method of proofing your bread dough, put the kneaded dough in a glass bowl and place it in the microwave. Put an 8-ounce glass of water in one corner of the microwave oven. As a beginning point, set the power level to 10%. Microwave for two minutes. If the dough feels hot (or put a yeast thermometer into the dough – it should never be over 112°F), allow the dough to rest in the oven for four minutes. If it does not feel hot but rather just cool to lukewarm, microwave it for an additional minute and allow it to rest for three minutes. Then microwave it again for two or three minutes (the same amount of time that you used before) and allow it to rest for six or seven minutes in the microwave. At the end of this time, the dough should feel comfortably warm, have doubled in volume, and an indentation should remain when poked with your finger. If it is not warm or has not doubled, try gradually increasing the power setting you use, but never go above 30%. If you use glass baking pans, the dough can be proofed in the microwave after shaping the loaf also.

If your dough felt hot after the first two minutes of microwaving on 10% power and does not rise properly, you should use the oven method (described on page 20) for proofing your dough.

Some microwave oven instruction manuals and cookbooks contain recipes for baking yeast breads in the microwave. I have not found this method to be satisfactory, mainly because breads baked in the microwave oven do not brown.

MIXERS

Any electric mixer can do at least part of the kneading required to make yeast bread; heavy-duty mixers can do all of the kneading for you. There are a number of mixers on the market that do a great job of doing all of the kneading by themselves. Kitchen Aid mixers are strong enough to develop gluten properly without any help from you and can make dough for two to four loaves of bread per batch depending on the capacity of the mixer bowl. They can be used to make two batches of dough in a row before you must allow your machine a 45 minute cool down period.

Kenwood mixers have a very powerful motor and a thermal overload protector so can be used to make as many batches of bread dough in a row as desired. The models with 7-quart bowls can be used to make dough for up to four loaves of bread at a time. However, you may have to stop and scrape the bowl during the initial mixing of bread dough to get all of the flour to mix in efficiently. For other foods (cookie dough, cakes, etc.) you may also find that Kenwood mixers are not especially efficient in getting all the ingredients well mixed without help from you.

Bosch mixers also have a powerful motor and a thermal overload protector, so they can be used to make an unlimited number of batches of dough consecutively. The large Bosch Universal mixer can make dough for five loaves of bread at a time. These mixers mix the flour in very efficiently and "clean the bowl" without assistance from you.

There are several advantages of using a mixer to make bread. One is that by using a large, heavy-duty mixer you can make several loaves at once and store them in your freezer to use as needed. Another advantage is that mixer-made breads have an excellent texture. Because you have an opportunity to check the consistency of the dough by hand, any variations in the amount of flour required because of weather, humidity, or flour quality can be corrected for.

See pages 47 and 51 for instructions on making yeast breads with a mixer.

FOOD PROCESSORS

A food processor is a piece of equipment that many of us already own which can be used to make yeast bread dough with gluten-containing flours. Food processors knead bread dough very quickly; in one minute they achieve excellent gluten development. You can use most processors to knead dough for only one loaf of bread at a time. The opportunity to check the dough by hand allows for the correction of any problems due to variations in the ingredients or weather. The texture of the bread is excellent. However, food processors cannot be used to make low gluten breads.

For instructions on using your food processor to make yeast breads, see pages 43 to 44.

BREAD MACHINES

Bread machines have revolutionized the lives of those of us who must make all of our bread ourselves because of our special diets. All we have to do is measure the ingredients and push a few buttons, and in a few hours we have bread! Several years ago, I had a bread baking day about every two weeks, baked six to ten loaves of various kinds of bread, and stocked up the freezer for the next two weeks. I enjoyed the feel of the dough and the aesthetic experience of making bread myself and was not an easy convert to bread machine baking, but now I could not live without my bread machines. They get more use than my washer and dryer. For those of us on special diets, a bread machine is not a luxury item, but rather is an essential time and energy saving appliance like a dishwasher or a clothes washer. To go back to making bread by hand now would be almost like digging out my grandmother's old washing board and tub to do laundry.

BREAD MACHINE FEATURES

There are many factors to consider when choosing a bread machine. Each bread machine has its own assets and drawbacks. Our needs and budgets are different, so there is no one machine that is best for every home baker. Some of the features that you should consider when making this important purchase are price, pan shape and size, viewing window, ease of keeping the machine clean, delayed cycle timer, programmability, the cycles the machine offers, and the power saver feature.

PRICE: This is probably the first factor that comes to mind when you are thinking about buying a bread machine. There are many economical models on the market now that do a great job of making ordinary breads without all the "bells and whistles" of the luxury machines. Also, most bread machines go on sale occasionally, so it is worth your while to shop around for a good price. Consider all of the features below and decide which of them you really need before you spend a lot of money for features you may rarely use.

PAN SHAPE AND SIZE: Most bread machines on the market now make either 1½ or 2 pound loaves. Since it is so easy to make bread with a bread machine and bread is best when freshly made, an individual or small family may be kept in bread adequately by a 1½ pound machine. I often run my machines more than once in a day, which is always a possibility with a smaller machine. For a large family, a large machine may be more practical. For one or two people, you might consider getting one of the new compact models which make 1 pound loaves.

Bread machine pans are most often vertically rectangular or horizontally rectangular. If you will be making mostly the more unusual types of breads which require assistance in the mixing and kneading parts of the cycle, you might consider getting a machine with a square bottom and a vertically rectangular pan because it may need less mixing help from you. However, a few machines with horizontally rectangular pans have two kneading bars; these machines mix and knead efficiently with little or no assistance from the cook.

Machines with horizontally rectangular pans produce loaves that look almost like store-bought, both as whole loaves and as slices. Machines with vertically rectangular pans produce square or tall rectangular slices depending on which direction you slice the bread.

VIEWING WINDOW: A viewing window is a good feature to have because it helps to keep an eye on how your bread is doing especially the first time you use a new recipe. When experimenting with unusual flours, being able to see what was going on and take action kept the dough from over-rising and running down over the edge of the pan and onto the heating coil of the machine more than once for me! But a viewing window is not an absolutely essential feature. If your machine does not have a window, you can lift the lid and take a few brief peeks to see what is happening. I have never had bread come out under-done or any of the other disasters that the manufacturers predict happen as a result of peeking into the machine.

DELAYED CYCLE TIMER: A timer is a useful feature to have if you want to have bread freshly baked for breakfast or for dinner when you will be away from home during the afternoon. Many machines with delayed cycle timers are called programmable but this may just mean that you can program what time you want your bread to be done, not that you have the control over the cycles that truly programmable machines, described below, give you. When deciding whether to get a machine with this feature, let your lifestyle and your budget be your guide.

PROGRAMMABILITY: If you want to make a variety of non-wheat breads, this is a very important feature for you to consider. In a non-programmable machine, you have one or a few set cycles to choose from. Wheat breads fit these cycles quite well; most of the spelt breads, kamut bread, and some rye breads can also be made using them. But if you wish to make some of the "variety" spelt-based breads, oat, barley, quinoa, amaranth, buckwheat, egg-free rice, or a number of other types of bread, you must have control over the final rising and baking times of the cycle to produce an acceptable loaf of bread. With a truly programmable machine, you can pre-program the kneading, rising, and baking times for one or more cycles and store these customized cycles in the memory of your machine. Be careful when purchasing a machine called "programmable" however. Often this only means that you can program the delayed cycle timer to have bread ready at a set time, not that you can control the lengths of various parts of the bread machine cycle.

There is one programmable machine on the market at the time of this writing, the Zojiruishi BBCC-V20. I recommend this machine even for bakers who are not cooking for a food allergy or gluten-free diet if the cost of the machine is not an issue. Since most of the questions I hear about bread machines are asked by allergy patients wondering how well a bread machine will meet their needs, this machine will be discussed in detail at the end of this chapter.

CRUST DARKNESS CONTROL: Some experienced bread machine bakers consider this feature essential. I personally almost always leave the darkness control on "medium" and do not use it. When I have tried using "light" for sweet breads, the crust has still come out too dark. This is not a feature that I would pay extra money for, although if the machine that you plan to get for other reasons has it, it is certainly not a drawback.

PRE-HEAT TIME AT THE BEGINNING OF THE CYCLE: Most bread machines have a pre-heat time at the beginning of their cycles which may be from about five to twenty minutes long. Unless you are planning to use cold water or put milk directly from the refrigerator into your machine, a long pre-heating time is not necessary. Just put the ingredients into the machine at somewhere near the correct temperature instead! However, neither is a long pre-heat a problem that should keep you from buying an otherwise desirable bread machine.

COOL DOWN OR KEEP WARM FEATURE AT THE END OF THE CYCLE: If you tend to get busy with other things and forget about your bread machine or if you want to leave home while it is running, a cool down feature is a very helpful feature to have. It will keep your bread from getting soggy if you do not remove it from the machine immediately. A keep warm feature keeps your bread warm and also keeps it from getting soggy if you do not remove it from the machine as soon as it finishes baking.

POWER SAVER FEATURE: Some bread machines have a backup system that keeps them from aborting the cycle during short power outages. The length of the outage the machine will allow varies widely. If your machine does not have this feature and a power outage occurs early in the cycle, you may be able to re-start the machine or you can pull the dough out of the machine, let it rise in a bread pan, and bake it in the oven. If you live in an area that has frequent short power outages, this feature may be important to you.

YEAST OR RAISIN DISPENSER: Some machines have a separate compartment to place the yeast in and the machine adds it to the dough after the cycle has begun. This can be an advantage when using your machine on the timer because there is no way that the yeast can get wet before it should. However, if you add the liquid ingredients to the machine first and put the yeast in a small well on top of the flour (even if you normally add ingredients to your machine in the opposite order), the yeast will stay dry without this feature.

A few machines have a raisin dispenser which adds raisins or nuts to your bread near the end of the kneading time. This feature is useful if you want to make raisin bread using the delayed cycle timer when you will be away from home, but if you rarely make raisin bread, it may not be worth spending extra money to get a raisin dispenser.

EASE OF KEEPING THE MACHINE CLEAN: Bread machines vary in how easy they are to keep clean. Most machines have pans which you remove from the machine before adding the ingredients. Some machines have crumb trays at the bottom of the machine or removable lids. I personally would choose a machine that worked well, even if it were not easy to keep clean, over one that was easier to keep clean but did not do what I wanted it to do, but this is an area where your personal neatness preference must help you decide which machine you prefer.

BREAD MACHINE CYCLES: Every bread machine has a **REGULAR, BASIC** or **WHITE BREAD CYCLE** which is designed for making white bread with wheat flour and active dry yeast. This cycle usually also works well for other types of bread, such as white spelt, and on many machines is even good for whole grain breads.

QUICK YEAST CYCLE: A quick yeast cycle allows you to use quick-rise yeast to make wheat breads more quickly than the basic cycles on a bread machine or to make bread with "instant" or even regular active dry yeast in a shorter amount of time, usually about two hours. On some machines, this cycle can be useful for making non-wheat yeast breads with regular active dry yeast because the second rising time is considerably shorter than in the regular cycles. However, on many machines the second rise may still be too long for some non-wheat flours that require a programmable cycle. This cycle is good for people in a hurry and for most machines produces excellent bread.

ONE-HOUR CYCLE: Some of the newer bread machines feature a cycle that makes a loaf of bread in about one hour. I have used the one-hour cycle on two machines, and while they certainly produce bread quickly, the quality of the bread is poor. The kneading time is insufficient, and you must compensate for the short rising time by using a very large quantity of yeast, usually four to six times as much as would normally be used. These factors produce a loaf of bread that may be dense and lacks the delicious flavor and texture expected from homemade bread. Many machines have quick rise cycles which make excellent bread in about two hours. Therefore, when choosing a bread machine, I consider a quick rise cycle preferable to a one-hour cycle.

WHOLE GRAIN CYCLE: If you plan to make a lot of 100% whole wheat bread, this can be a useful cycle on some machines. However, most machines have a fairly long basic yeast bread cycle with quite a bit of time devoted to kneading and a long second rise, so on many machines the whole grain cycle does not produce results that are substantially different from the standard cycle. If you are considering buying a bread machine for its whole grain cycle, consult the instruction booklet or the manufacturer for the times the machine spends on kneading and the second rise for both the standard and whole grain cycles and compare them to see if they are much different.

FRENCH BREAD CYCLE: This cycle is for dough that is low in fat and sugar and takes longer to rise. If you think that French and Italian breads should be long, crispy-crusted loaves rather than bread machine pan shaped loaves, you may prefer to make French bread by using the dough cycle, shaping the loaves on baking sheets, brushing the crust with egg white or bread or bun wash (see the recipe on page 111) to make it crispy, and baking your French or Italian bread the oven. You can produce much better French and Italian bread by this method than by purchasing a machine with a French bread cycle.

SWEET BREAD CYCLE: A sweet bread cycle allows the dough more rising time and bakes it at a lower temperature than the standard cycle does. Even when the sweet bread cycle is used, I still find that the crust of sweet breads baked in the machine is darker than I prefer. Instead of using the sweet bread cycle to make sweet breads, I use the dough cycle, shape the dough, and bake the bread in the oven, where it is easier to control how dark the crust will get.

RAISIN BREAD CYCLE: A raisin bread cycle is usually a standard cycle with a "beep" to tell you when to add raisins or nuts to your bread machine so they do not get mashed by the full kneading cycle. Once you know how long your machine kneads on the standard cycle, you can set your kitchen timer for about five minutes before the last kneading time should be finished when you start the machine and add the raisins or nuts when the timer rings. Therefore, while helpful, this is not an essential bread machine feature. Many machines, rather than having a special raisin bread cycle, include a "beep" which tells you when to add raisins or nuts on many of the cycles.

DOUGH CYCLE: A bread machine with a dough cycle feature makes the dough and allows it to rise, and then stops the machine before baking so you can shape and bake the dough as you desire. Some of the cheaper machines claim to have a dough cycle, but what they really have is a buzzer that tells you when to remove the dough from the machine if you do not want it to be baked. If you are not at home or are not paying attention to your machine, it may bake your dough before you notice it. With any machine, you can set a timer to remind you to stop the machine before it bakes, but a dough cycle that turns the machine off for you is a very useful feature to have if you want to have dough ready to make into rolls or pizza for dinner when you are not going to be home in the afternoon.

BAKE-ONLY CYCLE: If you plan to use your machine to occasionally make low-gluten bread, a bake-only cycle will allow you to do it successfully without spending the money for a programmable machine. You can use the dough cycle, allow the bread to raise the proper length of time for its second rise, and then stop the dough cycle and start the bake-only cycle. However, you will have to be present at the right time to do this.

QUICK BREAD (NON-YEAST) OR CAKE CYCLE: This cycle is essential if you are allergic to yeast or want to make non-yeast quick breads or cakes in your bread machine. It is most useful for people who need to eat yeast-free breads because of food allergies or who are on a low-yeast diet for *Candida* control. If you are considering buying a machine for the quick bread cycle, be sure to check the chart in the instruction book which says how long each part of the cycles last. Some machines have a quick bread cycle with a very long initial mixing time before baking. The ideal mixing time for the recipes in this book is three to four minutes of fast mixing. (This may follow a minute or two of slow mixing). If the machine you wish to purchase mixes a little longer than this, it is still usable (see instructions on page 19) but if it mixes for fifteen minutes and you plan to use the quick bread cycle often, I would suggest choosing another machine.

If you want a bread machine mostly for making yeast breads and rarely make non-yeast breads, a quick bread cycle may not be essential for you because quick breads are very easy to make by hand. When deciding on this feature, let your dietary needs, your budget, and how much you plan to make quick breads be your guide.

THE QUESTION I am most often asked is "Which bread machine should I buy?" The answer varies from year to year and sometimes even from month to month. Like automobile manufacturers, bread machine manufacturers change their products often. Also, the needs of each home baker are different. Ask yourself what you need: Will you be away from home and want to come home to a freshly baked loaf of bread to go with your dinner? Then get a machine with a delayed cycle timer. How much bread will you or your family eat? How often do you want to bake? If you have a large family or do not want to bake every day or two, get a larger capacity machine. Do you have frequent power outages in your area? How long do the outages last? How much do you expect to use your machine? How much money can you afford to spend on it? How much money will it save you?

For people who must eat special breads, such as those on food allergy diets, the last question is crucial. If by making your own bread you will eliminate the weekly necessity of buying two or three small loaves of expensive frozen bread from the health food store, paying a little more for a bread machine is justified.

The most important bread machine feature for making non-wheat breads is the ability to control the length of the last rising time before the bread bakes. There are two options for this. The "cheaper" choice is to buy a machine with a bake-only cycle and a dough cycle that includes rising time as well as mixing time. Then use the dough cycle followed by the bake-only cycle to make your special bread as described in the bake-only cycle section above. Bake-only cycles are not uncommon, and many economical machines can be used to make special breads in this way.

The option for controlling the last rising time that is "more expensive" in terms of initial investment is to buy a truly programmable machine. As with all bread machines, programmable models change frequently. Zojirushi was the first to introduce a truly programmable machine in the early 1990's with their $350 BBCC-S15 model, and they have continued to make excellent programmable machines. My current favorite and the machine I use several times a week is the Zojirushi Home Baker model BBCC-V20 which cost me about $150. This 2-pound machine has a horizontally rectangular pan with two kneading bars and makes large normal-shaped loaves of bread. The two kneading bars produce a mixing motion that includes both ends of the pan, so for most types of bread, the cook does not have to make sure that all the flour in the corners of the pan has been incorporated into the loaf. This machine's standard cycles including basic, whole grain, dough, quick basic, quick whole grain, and quick dough cycles, a cake (non-yeast) cycle, a jam cycle, a signal to add raisins for raisin bread on most of the cycles, and a "homemade menu" programmable cycle. The "homemade menu" cycle can be programmed right before baking, so if you have more than one special cycle that you want to use regularly, it is easy to change the menu before making a loaf of bread. The quick yeast bread cycles on this machine make excellent bread using SAF™ instant yeast in about two hours. The quick dough cycle only takes 45 minutes. I most often use the quick cycles to make wheat or white spelt bread or dough. This machine is a very "mellow" kneader and produces excellent spelt bread as a result.

The up-and-coming programmable Zojirushi machine is the Home Baker model BBCC-X20 which costs about $200. This machine can be programmed with three special "homemade menu" cycles, has a shorter warm-up time than the BBCC-V20 on the standard cycles, and is otherwise very similar to the Zojirushi BBCC-V20.

Although Breadman machines are wonderful for making wheat bread, their truly programmable Breadman Ultimate model kneads the dough very vigorously, almost violently, which overdevelops the gluten in spelt bread. The extreme kneading also is less-than-ideal for low-gluten breads recipes that depend on guar or xanthum gum to give the dough structure. However, if you are planning to make only wheat bread, Breadman machines are fairly economical, have many options, and make great bread.

For people who do not have allergies or gluten intolerance and plan to make wheat bread most of the time, an economical machine will probably fit your needs. For an expenditure of less than $100 you can enjoy fresh homemade bread as often as you like.

THE CHOICE is yours. At an allergy cooking class I was recently asked, "Do you have any recommendations for people who are on a special diet and don't want to spend a lot of time cooking?" My immediate reply was, "Get a bread machine." If you are on a special diet, a bread machine can save you a lot of time and energy. When you are planning to buy a bread machine, get information about the machines you are considering from the manufacturers. Go to stores and look at bread machines and the instruction booklets that come with them. Check the details of the cycles by reading the cycle time charts which are sometimes included in the instruction booklets. Shop around for sales, and get the machine that best serves your needs for the lowest price. Then enjoy your homemade bread and the time you do not have to spend making it.

The Building Blocks of Bread

Just as we are what we eat, our bread is as good as what we put into it. One of the greatest advantages of making your own bread is that you control what goes into it. You can put in the freshest, most wholesome ingredients and leave out the preservatives and chemicals that are found in many commercial breads. Knowing what ingredients you can use to build your bread and using the best ingredients available will help you turn out delicious, nutritious loaves every time.

FLOURS

Flour is the most basic building block of bread. For all yeast breads, but especially if you are using a bread machine, it is essential that you use good quality flour. When you are making bread in a bread machine, it is also essential that you measure accurately if you want your bread to turn out well every time.

Flour does not need to be sifted before measuring when you are making bread. Simply stir it to loosen it, lightly spoon it into your measuring cup, and level it off with a straight-edged knife or spatula. Resist the temptation to pack flour into the cup or a heavy, dry loaf of bread may result. Even with the best flour there can be many variables such as the moisture and gluten content. When making bread by hand these variables are corrected for by adding flour until the bread "feels right." With a bread machine, you will learn to judge the bread by how it looks and by reaching into the machine and checking how it feels. "Right" for bread machine bread is usually softer than "right" for bread made by hand. Also, for some types of flour such as rye, the right texture of the dough is quite sticky.

Some people grind their own flour from whole grains in order to make fresher, better tasting, more economical, and more nutritious bread. Home ground flours are delicious but can be more variable than commercial flour because we cannot test and blend the flour for gluten content, etc., before we use it. If you are a beginning bread maker or are just getting used to using a bread machine, it may be best to start with high quality, reliable commercial flour until you learn the right feel of the dough. Then, after you have gained some experience, you will be able to judge the dough and compensate for variations in your home ground flour by using slightly more or less flour or liquid.

THE KINDS OF FLOUR USED IN THE RECIPES IN THIS BOOK INCLUDE:

BREAD FLOUR is wheat flour made from high-gluten wheat. The higher gluten content of this flour makes it perfect for bread machine breads. The bran and germ have been removed from bread flour, and some brands are bleached and bromated. Bread flour from King Arthur Flour Company (see "Sources," page 211) is an excellent bread flour that has not been chemically treated. If you live in an area of the country where you can get King Arthur flour easily, it will consistently give you excellent results in your bread machine. If you use a national brand of flour, be aware that not all bread flour works equally well all of the time. One national brand I used when I first got a bread machine usually worked well, but then I got a few bags that made flat-topped, fallen loaves of bread until I began adding vital gluten to my bread. I switched to a different national brand. The next time the first brand of flour was on sale I tried it again, and it worked well. In the intervening years I have had short-term problems with both of these national brands of flour.

ALL PURPOSE FLOUR or **UNBLEACHED FLOUR** is refined wheat flour that is lower in gluten content than bread flour. These types of flour are used in the quick bread recipes in this book. They may be used for making yeast breads by hand, but will require that more flour be added to the recipe than if bread flour is used. All purpose flour and unbleached flour are not recommended for making yeast breads using a bread machine.

WHOLE WHEAT BREAD FLOUR is whole wheat flour that has been ground from hard red spring or winter wheat and is higher in gluten than most whole wheat flour. (Graham flour is whole wheat flour ground from low-gluten wheat). If you use whole wheat bread flour in your bread machine rather than regular whole wheat flour, it will make breads that rise well even though they are 100% whole grain. King Arthur Flour and Arrowhead Mills produce excellent whole wheat bread flour.

WHOLE WHEAT ALL PURPOSE FLOUR is whole wheat flour that is lower in gluten than whole wheat bread flour. It is used in quick breads in this book. It can be used in whole wheat yeast breads with good results by also using the optional vital gluten called for in the whole wheat bread recipes.

WHITE WHOLE WHEAT FLOUR is milled from hard white wheat. It is lighter in flavor and color than whole wheat bread flour and so may be more acceptable to people who are not whole grain enthusiasts. King Arthur Flour offers a great white whole wheat flour which makes excellent bread. (See "Sources," page 211).

GLUTEN FLOUR is a refined wheat flour that is about 40 to 50% gluten. It is very high in protein, and is often used by hypoglycemics. It can be used to "fix" low quality flours by adding more gluten to the recipe. Use about ¼ cup gluten flour and ¾ cup of the other flour for each cup of flour called for in the recipe.

VITAL GLUTEN is refined wheat flour that has had the starch removed and is almost all gluten. It is commonly used to "fix" low quality flours and to make dense breads rise better. However, if you use it to make non-wheat breads rise better, the bread will no longer be wheat-free, because vital gluten comes from wheat. If you are using it to improve your results with whole wheat flour, use 2 to 4 teaspoons for a small loaf of bread and up to 2 tablespoons for a large loaf. Vital gluten is given as an optional ingredient in a few whole wheat bread recipes in this book. However, if you use good quality whole wheat bread flour, your bread will turn out well without the vital gluten.

WHOLE SPELT FLOUR: Spelt is a grain that is closely related to wheat and is higher in gluten than wheat. (Spelt and wheat are in the same biological genus but different species. See page 217 for more information about the confusion about the relationship between spelt and wheat). Spelt makes excellent bread, but I have found more variability between types of spelt flour than for any other kind of flour. Even the best spelt flour can vary from bag to bag, so always test the consistency of the dough as described on page 56 when you start a loaf of spelt bread in your machine. The only brand of spelt flour I have used that consistently produces excellent bread is Purity Foods spelt flour. (See "Sources," page 212). Purity Foods flour is milled from a European strain of spelt that is higher in protein and gluten than most spelt. All of the spelt recipes in this book were developed using Purity Foods flour.

WHITE SPELT FLOUR is whole spelt flour that has been sifted, removing the fibrous elements of the grain, but not bleached, bromated, or enriched like refined wheat flour usually is. It is available only from Purity Foods. (See "Sources," page 212). It is the best non-wheat flour for making non-wheat breads in a bread machine, and produces light, fluffy breads that are almost impossible to distinguish from wheat breads. As with whole spelt flour, always test the consistency of the dough as described on page 56 when you start your bread to compensate for variations in the flour.

KAMUT FLOUR: Kamut is another grain that is closely related to wheat. Although the gluten structure it forms in yeast bread is not as strong as wheat's structure, it still produces very good bread. It is golden yellow in color and has a flavor very similar to wheat. Kamut breads made without a bread machine need only one rising time. After you make the dough, shape it and put it in loaf pans immediately, and bake it after it rises once.

RYE FLOUR is a gluten-containing flour, although it is lower in gluten than wheat. Whole grain rye flour produces dense but very flavorful breads. I have occasionally found that rye flour from health food store bulk bins made bread that did not rise properly. Arrowhead Mills rye flour produces rye flour that makes consistently good bread.

WHITE RYE FLOUR is rye flour with the bran and germ removed. Lighter bread can be made from white rye flour than from whole rye flour. It is also a good choice for those on low fiber diets. White rye flour is available from the King Arthur Flour Baker's Catalogue. (See "Sources," page 211).

BROWN RICE FLOUR is milled from the whole rice grain and contains the rice polish, bran, and germ. It is a gluten-free flour and is acceptable on celiac diets. Bread made from rice flour usually contains ingredients to strengthen the bread's structure such as eggs. Egg-free rice bread can be made by hand or in a programmable bread machine by using guar gum to strengthen the structure of the bread.

WHITE RICE FLOUR is milled from rice that has been polished so the fibrous portions of the grain have been removed. White rice flour is a good bread ingredient for those on low fiber diets. Like brown rice flour, it is also gluten-free and acceptable on celiac diets.

BARLEY FLOUR is a low-gluten flour. If you wish to make bread from only barley flour in a bread machine, you will need a programmable machine because the structure of barley bread is fragile. If it rises for a standard amount of time, it will collapse during baking.

OAT FLOUR is also a low-gluten flour. As with barley, a programmable machine is necessary to make good oat-only machine-made yeast bread. Oats are an excellent source of soluble fiber.

CORN MEAL gives bread an interesting texture and a sweet flavor. It is gluten-free and is acceptable on celiac diets. Corn cannot be used alone to make yeast bread, but masa harina, a specially processed corn flour, makes excellent tortillas. If you cannot find masa harina locally, see "Sources," page 212, for ordering information.

SOY FLOUR is ground from soybeans. It is very high in protein, and may be used to increase the protein content of breads. It is acceptable on celiac diets.

CAROB POWDER is a substitute for cocoa on allergy diets. Added to pumpernickel bread, it gives a rich brown color.

AMARANTH FLOUR is a non-grain flour that is quite useful to people who are allergic to all grains. It is good tasting, very nutritious, and high in protein, but I have encountered problems with stickiness with amaranth flour more often than with any other kind of flour I have used. However, since there have been times in my life when amaranth was the only flour I could eat, I persisted in using it, and if my bread came out sticky, I sliced and toasted it. Amaranth flour makes very dense bread. Purchase it from a store that either has a high turnover or refrigerates its flour and store it in the refrigerator or freezer at home or it may develop a strong flavor.

QUINOA FLOUR is also a non-grain flour which is related to beets and spinach. It is high in protein and calcium and is very nutritious. It has a distinctive flavor, and is best in breads that contain fruit, which moderates the flavor. Quinoa breads are very dense.

BUCKWHEAT FLOUR is a non-grain flour. Dark buckwheat flour is ground from roasted buckwheat groats. Arrowhead Mills produces an excellent dark buckwheat flour that consistently makes good bread. White buckwheat flour is ground from unroasted groats and has a milder flavor. Commercial white buckwheat flour can vary tremendously from bag to bag, even from the same source. White buckwheat flour is often home ground. If you wish to make bread from white buckwheat flour, make a loaf or two of regular buckwheat bread with Arrowhead Mills flour first to gain experience with what the consistency of buckwheat bread dough should be. Then make bread with white buckwheat flour using the same recipe and, if necessary, adding more flour to reach the same consistency. You can often substitute white buckwheat flour for dark buckwheat flour in equal amounts.

GARBANZO and **TEFF FLOURS** are used only in tortilla recipes in this book. Teff, and also milo and millet, are non-gluten grains that are great additions to the diets of people with food allergies, but they yield such fragile baked goods that they are not suitable for bread machine baking. Garbanzo flour is ground from garbanzo beans and is unrelated to grains. For more recipes made with these and even more "exotic" wheat and grain substitutes, refer to *The Ultimate Food Allergy Cookbook and Survival Guide* as described on the last pages of this book.

TAPIOCA FLOUR, also called tapioca starch or tapioca starch flour, is a white starch that is an excellent addition to gluten-free or low-gluten breads. It strengthens the structure of these breads and allows them to rise better.

ARROWROOT is a white starch that looks much like cornstarch and may be used in place of tapioca flour to strengthen the structure of gluten-free breads.

POTATO FLOUR: Potato flour and potato starch are not the same thing. The recipes in this book use potato flour, which is a less refined flour, rather than potato starch. Potato flour is a useful addition to gluten-free rice breads. Bob's Red Mill produces good potato flour. (See "Sources," page 212).

LEAVENING INGREDIENTS

Leavening is due to gas produced by yeast or by acidic and basic ingredients that, when combined, yield gas which causes non-yeast bread to rise. There are several varieties of yeast that you can use to make bread by hand or in your bread machine. Non-yeast breads are leavened by baking soda plus an acid ingredient. Both the acidic and basic components are "built in" to baking powder, or you can use baking soda plus any of a variety of acid ingredients. The leavening ingredients used in this book include:

ACTIVE DRY YEAST: Active dry yeast is yeast that has been freeze-dried to retain its activity. An expiration date is usually stamped on the package, and the yeast should work well until that date if you store it in the refrigerator after opening it. Active dry yeast is available in ¼ ounce (2¼ teaspoon) packets or 4 ounce jars in most grocery stores. Also, you can purchase it in one or two pound bags and store the yeast in your freezer. Do not repeatedly thaw and refreeze the bag of yeast, but rather occasionally take out a small amount to use within a few weeks. Keep the yeast you removed from the bag in a jar in your refrigerator and return the bag to the freezer before the yeast has time to thaw. I have had consistently good results using Red Star™ active dry yeast in my bread machines.

INSTANT, BREAD MACHINE, OR QUICK-RISE YEAST: Although the recipes in this book do not call for these types of yeast, you may wish to use them to save time. If you are making bread with a good gluten structure, you can add the same amount of these types of yeast as of active dry yeast to produce a higher, lighter loaf. (However, the first time you do this with each recipe, watch your bread machine to make sure the dough is not going to run over the edge of the pan). If your loaf is too large when made with quick-rise yeast, you may decrease the amount of yeast used by about one fourth to produce a more normal sized loaf. Quick-rise yeast can be used to make wheat-containing breads more quickly using the quick yeast cycle on some bread machines, or to make breads that rise more quickly by hand. Instant, bread machine, and quick-rise yeast are not recommended for non-wheat bread machine breads because their gluten structure is more fragile; if these yeasts are used, the bread may over-rise and then collapse during baking.

SAF Red™ instant yeast is my favorite yeast for baking white bread using the "quick yeast" cycle of my bread machine. However, I live at relatively high altitude (about 5500 feet). The King Arthur Flour Company recommends SAF™ instant yeast for use with the quick-rise cycle of the Zojirushi Home Bakery in general (with no reference to altitude) but my son, who lives near sea level, finds that SAF Red™ works well with the regular cycle and produces dense bread with the quick rise cycle. You may have to experiment with SAF™ and the various cycles on your machine to see what works for you. At high altitude I use SAF™ only for white or mostly-white bread made with bread flour. I use active dry yeast for whole wheat and non-wheat breads, including white spelt bread, and routinely use the quick-rise cycles on my Zojirushi Home Bakery to make whole wheat, whole spelt, and white spelt bread.

SAF Red™ comes in one pound bags that usually cost just a dollar or so more than the price of a 4 ounce jar of active dry yeast. If you can buy it locally at your health food store, SAF™ is very economical to use. It is also available by mail-order from King Arthur Flour (See "Sources," page 211) and even with the shipping charges, it is still a bargain. Store most of the package in your freezer, put just enough for a few weeks' baking in your refrigerator, and you can use one package for a long time.

YEAST FOR SWEET OR ACID BREADS is also available from King Arthur Flour. SAF Gold™ Instant Yeast is wonderful for breads that are acidic, such as sourdough, or high in sweeteners. When made with active dry or "regular" instant yeast, these types of bread can take a long time to rise; with SAF Gold™ the rising time is not prolonged. SAF Gold™ comes in bags that weigh just under one pound.

BAKING POWDER: The quick breads in this book are leavened by baking powder, either alone or with baking soda. Baking powder is used in all of the bread machine quick bread recipes in this book because it can withstand the longer mixing times that the machines use without exhausting all of its leavening power. Baking powder is a combination of baking soda, an acid ingredient, and a starch. Some baking powders contain aluminum, which probably should be avoided for good health. Rumford™ baking powder is aluminum-free and contains cornstarch. If you must avoid cornstarch because of a corn allergy, Featherweight™ baking powder contains potato starch and is aluminum-free.

BAKING SODA: Baking soda is used with any of a variety of acid ingredients to produce leavening in handmade quick breads. If you are making non-yeast bread by hand with baking soda and an acid ingredient rather than baking powder, be sure to work quickly so the leavening activity is not exhausted before the bread goes into the oven. (For more about this, see pages 18 to 19). Baking soda is used along with baking powder in some of this book's bread machine quick bread recipes which contain acidic fruits.

SWEETNERS

FRUIT JUICE CONCENTRATES which are purchased frozen are used extensively in the recipes in this book. Yeast grows best when it has some sugar to nourish it, and the fruit sugar in fruit juice concentrates is a healthy food for both yeast and people. If you bake bread that requires fruit juice concentrate often, you may wish to keep a can of apple juice concentrate in your refrigerator so it is always thawed and ready to use in breads.

Many of the recipes in this book use apple juice concentrate as a sweetener. If you are allergic to apples, you can use another fruit juice concentrate, such as pineapple juice concentrate. Or you can use a juice, such as white grape juice. To use a juice (not a concentrate), use four times the amount of juice as the amount of apple juice concentrate the recipe calls for and decrease the water by three times the volume of apple juice concentrate the recipe calls for. For example, if you want to use white grape juice to make a 1½ pound loaf of white corn bread (recipe on page 68), you would use 1 cup of grape juice (this amount is four times the ¼ cup of apple juice concentrate called for) and ⅛ cup water (this is the ⅞ cup water called for minus ¾ cup which is three times the amount of apple juice concentrate called for). The total amount (volume) of liquid must stay the same. In this example, for the original recipe:

¼ cup apple juice concentrate + ⅞ cup water = 1⅛ cup liquid.

After making the substitution:

1 cup white grape juice + ⅛ cup water = 1⅛ cup liquid.

FRUIT SWEET™, GRAPE SWEET™, AND PEAR SWEET™ are more concentrated fruit juice sweeteners than frozen fruit juice concentrates and can be used interchangeably in the recipes in this book. Fruit Sweet™ is a combination of peach, pear, and pineapple juice concentrates. Grape Sweet™ is made from grape juice concentrate. Pear Sweet™ is made from pear juice concentrate. All three are useful in sweet breads where more sweetness is desired than can be added with regular fruit juice concentrates. If too much of these or other fruit sweeteners is used in yeast breads, the acidity of the sweetener can inhibit the growth of the yeast causing very slow rising. Substituting SAF Gold™ yeast for active dry yeast can help overcome this problem.

DATE SUGAR is ground dried dates. It is useful both in sweet bread doughs and as a sweetener you can sprinkle, such as in the filling for cinnamon rolls.

HONEY is a sweeter-tasting and more concentrated sweetener than the fruit sweeteners above. It also has a more profound effect on blood sugar levels, and may not be tolerated by hypoglycemics and allergy patients with candidiasis. It is used as an optional alternative ingredient to fruit sweeteners in some of the recipes in this book where more sweetness may be desired.

FATS

OIL is used in minimal amounts in most of the bread recipes in this book. Fats make bread tender and keep it from becoming stale rapidly.

LECITHIN: Liquid lecithin is included as an optional ingredient in most of the recipes in this book because it is very effective at keeping bread from getting dry and adds moistness to the bread more effectively than oil. It is also said to be a dough conditioner and promote higher rising although I have not noticed that it makes much difference in this regard. Liquid lecithin is very sticky but it can be easily measured by measuring the oil first and then using the same spoon to measure the lecithin.

MISCELLANEOUS INGREDIENTS

SALT is a very important ingredient in yeast breads. It moderates the growth of the yeast and prevents over-proofing which can lead to the bread collapsing when it is baked. It strengthens the gluten structure of the bread by inhibiting enzymes in the flour that break gluten down. Salt also adds flavor to bread. A few salt-free recipes made with bread flour and white spelt flour are included in this book, but for most breads, especially those that do not have strong structures, it works much better to decrease the amount of salt used than to omit it entirely if you are on a low salt diet.

EGGS strengthen the structure of breads and are especially important in gluten-free breads. The recipes in this book call for extra large eggs. If your eggs do not measure ¼ cup each, add a little water to bring them up to ¼ cup volume. Bring the eggs to room temperature and beat them slightly before adding them to your bread. If you forget to take them out of the refrigerator to warm up ahead of baking time, immerse them in a bowl of warm tap water for a few minutes to warm them up quickly.

EGG SUBSTITUTES such as Egg Beaters™ may be used in place of eggs in the few recipes in this book that call for eggs. By using them, you avoid eating the cholesterol that eggs contain. However, egg substitutes contain eggs whites and can contain milk or milk derivatives, corn derivatives, and wheat gluten, so they are not a good choice for people with food allergies. They are available refrigerated or frozen and may be frozen at home.

GUAR GUM is a soluble fiber that comes from a legume. It is used to impart structure to trap the leavening gas in gluten-free and low-gluten breads. Guar gum mixes readily with water and can be used interchangeably with xanthum gum. Guar gum is more economical than xanthum gum.

XANTHUM GUM is another soluble fiber that can be used to give structure to low-gluten and gluten-free breads. It comes from a bacteria, *Xanthomonas compestris*. It can be substituted for guar gum in the recipes in this book. If your bread comes out very dense, you may wish to increase the amount of guar or xanthum gum used by one-fourth to one-half. Xanthum gum does not mix readily with water, so to use it, mix it with part of the flour.

VITAMIN C CRYSTALS impart acid to yeast bread dough, which can strengthen the protein structure when used in moderation. It can also be used as the acid leavening component in handmade non-yeast breads. Vitamin C crystals and powder may be used interchangeably. Be sure whatever kind of vitamin C you use is unbuffered (does not contain minerals such as calcium or magnesium) or it will not impart acid to your bread.

BREAD FLAVORINGS such as Heidelberg rye sour and instant sourdough flavor can be purchased from King Arthur Flour. (See "Sources," page 211). They make it possible to imitate the flavor of sourdough bread without expending the time and effort of maintaining a starter and going through the process of making "real" sourdough. King Arthur also carries Lalvain du Jour™ freeze-dried sourdough starters which are added to the bread in small amounts along with regular yeast. These starters still require a multi-day process to make bread, but you do not have to maintain a starter.

RAISINS AND OTHER DRIED FRUITS, NUTS, SEEDS, AND GRAINS OR GRAIN COMPONENTS, such as cracked wheat, cracked spelt, wheat germ, oat bran, and oatmeal are used in some of the recipes in this book to provide extra fiber and a variety of textures and tastes.

Instructions and Recipes for
Food Processor and Mixer Yeast Breads
and Handmade Quick Breads

If you are not ready to purchase a bread machine, you can still use appliances that you may already have to save yourself time and effort when you make bread. A microwave oven can be used to make your bread rise in a fraction of the time it would normally take. (See pages 24 to 25). An electric mixer can do part or, if it is heavy-duty, all of the work of kneading bread for you, making several loaves at a time. And a food processor can knead the dough for a loaf of bread in just one minute.

Any of the bread machine recipes in this book can be made by hand or with your mixer. The recipes made with flours that contain a fair amount of gluten, such as wheat, spelt, and kamut, can also be made using a food processor. Breads made by hand or with a mixer or processor may absorb slightly more flour in the kneading process than bread machine breads take, so plan to use a little more flour. If you are using your food processor to make the dough, instead of increasing the flour, decrease the amount of the water in the bread machine recipe by about one-eighth cup (two tablespoons) to produce bread of the right consistency which will be slightly firmer than bread machine bread. Since you can add flour until the "feel" of the dough is right (see page 22), variations in the amount of moisture the flour contains, gluten content, etc. will be compensated for, so accurate measuring is not as critical as with bread machine breads. When making bread by hand or with one of these appliances, the most important factor is how the dough feels when the right amount of flour has been added and the gluten is properly developed. This is discussed more on page 56 and is something that you will learn with experience.

Instructions are given below for making yeast breads using a food processor or mixer and quick breads by hand. Some sample recipes are also included to guide you as you use the bread machine recipes in the following chapters to make bread by hand, mixer, or processor.

FOOD PROCESSOR BREADS

You can use a food processor to make dough for one loaf of bread at a time. Place the dough blade or metal blade used for pureeing into the machine. Put the dry ingredients, such as the flour, yeast, salt, dry sweeteners, and spices, in the processor bowl and pulse a few times to mix. Add the oil and lecithin (if you are using it) and pulse a few times until it is absorbed evenly by the flour. Combine the liquid ingredients such as water and fruit juice in a cup or bowl. They should be at or slightly above room temperature, about 80°F. Turn the processor on and add the liquid ingredients slowly through the feed tube, reserving about 1 tablespoon of liquid. When the dough forms a ball that cleans the side of the bowl (although there may be a few scraps of dough that do not join the ball), begin timing and process for one minute. Add the last tablespoon of liquid if necessary to make the dough form a ball. If the full amount of liquid does not make the dough form a ball, add an additional tablespoon of water. After the dough has kneaded for one minute, remove it from the processor and knead it briefly by hand on a floured board to check its consistency. If it is too sticky, knead in an additional 1 to 2 tablespoons of flour by hand. When you've added all the flour required, knead in raisins or nuts by hand. Put the dough in an oiled bowl, turn it over, and allow it to rise in a warm (85 to 90°F) place until doubled in volume, about 40 minutes to 1 hour. Or use your microwave oven to proof it as on pages 24 to 25. Punch the dough down and shape it into loaves or rolls as desired. (For loaves, use an 8-inch by 4-inch or 9-inch by 5-inch oiled loaf pan). Allow it to rise until double again. Bake loaves at 350°F to 375°F, usually for 45 minutes to an hour, and rolls at 375°F for 15 to 25 minutes.

Food Processor White Bread

3⅛ cups bread flour
1¾ teaspoons active dry or quick-rise yeast
1 teaspoon salt
1 tablespoons oil
½ tablespoon liquid lecithin or additional oil
2 tablespoons Fruit Sweet™ or honey
⅞ cup water or milk at room temperature

Prepare the dough as in the food processor bread directions on pages 43 and 44 and let it rise once. Punch down the dough and shape it into one loaf. Put it into an oiled loaf pan. Let it rise until it has doubled again, about 45 minutes if made with active dry yeast. Bake at 375°F for 40 to 45 minutes. Immediately remove it from the pan and cool it on a wire rack. Makes 1 loaf. This dough can also be used to make rolls or buns (pages 112 to 120), pizza (page 154), breadsticks (page 158), or pretzels (page 160). The nutritional analysis for this recipe is about the same as for a large loaf of "White Bread," page 60.

Food Processor White Spelt Bread

2⅞ cups white spelt flour
1¾ teaspoons active dry or quick-rise yeast
¾ teaspoon salt
2½ teaspoons oil
1 teaspoon liquid lecithin or additional oil
3 tablespoons apple juice concentrate at room temperature
⅝ cup water at room temperature

Prepare the dough as in the food processor bread directions on pages 43 and 44 and let it rise once. Punch down the dough and shape it into one loaf. Put it into an oiled loaf pan. Let it rise until it has doubled again, about 40 to 45 minutes if made with active dry yeast. Bake at 375°F for 40 to 45 minutes. Immediately remove it from the pan and cool it on a wire rack. Makes 1 loaf. This dough can also be used to make rolls or buns (pages 112 to 120), pizza (page 155), breadsticks (page 158), or pretzels (page 160). The nutritional analysis for this recipe is the same as for a large loaf of "White Spelt Bread," page 61.

Food Processor Whole Wheat Bread

3 cups whole wheat bread flour
1¾ teaspoon active dry or quick-rise yeast
¾ teaspoon salt
1 tablespoon oil
1 teaspoon liquid lecithin or additional oil
3 tablespoons apple juice concentrate at room temperature
1 cup water at room temperature

Prepare the dough as in the food processor bread directions on pages 43 and 44 and let it rise once. Punch down the dough and shape it into one loaf. Put it into an oiled loaf pan. Let it rise until it has doubled again, about 45 minutes if made with active dry yeast. Bake at 375°F for 40 to 45 minutes. Immediately remove it from the pan and cool it on a wire rack. Makes 1 loaf. This dough can also be used to make rolls or buns (pages 112 to 120), pizza (page 154), breadsticks (page 158), or pretzels (page 160). The nutritional analysis for this recipe is the same as for a small loaf of "100% Whole Wheat Bread," page 74.

Food Processor Whole Spelt Bread

3⅓ cups whole spelt flour
2¼ teaspoons active dry or quick-rise yeast
¾ teaspoon salt
1 tablespoon oil
½ tablespoon liquid lecithin or additional oil
¼ cup apple juice concentrate at room temperature
⅞ cup water at room temperature

Prepare the dough as in the food processor bread directions on pages 43 and 44 and let it rise once. Punch down the dough and shape it into one loaf. Put it into an oiled loaf pan. (This bread can be difficult to remove from the pan after baking, especially if you have baked it for the full baking time. If you prefer your bread well browned, also line the pan with oiled waxed or parchment paper). Let it rise until it has doubled again, about 40 to 45 minutes if made with active dry yeast. Bake at 375°F for 40 to 45 minutes. Immediately remove it from the pan and cool it on a wire rack. Makes 1 loaf. This dough can also be used to make rolls or buns (pages 112 to 120), pizza (page 154), breadsticks (page 158), or pretzels (page 160). The nutritional analysis for this recipe is the same as for a large loaf of "Whole Grain Spelt Bread," page 76.

Food Processor Kamut Bread

2¼ teaspoons active dry or quick-rise yeast
3¼ cup kamut flour
¾ teaspoons salt
2 tablespoons oil
¼ cup apple or pineapple juice concentrate at room temperature
1⅛ cups water at room temperature

Prepare the dough as in the food processor bread directions on pages 43 and 44 except do not let it rise the first time. After checking its consistency, shape it into a loaf and put it into an oiled loaf pan. Let it rise until it has doubled, about 45 minutes if made with active dry yeast. Bake at 375°F for 40 to 45 minutes. Immediately remove it from the pan and cool it on a wire rack. Makes 1 loaf. This dough can also be used to make rolls or buns (pages 112 to 120), pizza (page 154), breadsticks (page 158), or pretzels (page 160). The nutritional analysis for this recipe is the same as for a small loaf of "Kamut Bread," page 84.

MIXER BREADS MADE WITH HIGH-GLUTEN FLOURS

To make yeast bread using high-gluten flours such as wheat, spelt, kamut, or rye with your mixer, put one-half to two-thirds of the flour, the yeast, the salt, and the other dry ingredients in the mixer bowl. Mix on low speed for about 30 seconds. Warm the liquid ingredients to 115 to 120°F. With the mixer running on low speed, add the liquids to the dry ingredients in a slow stream. Continue mixing until the dry and liquid ingredients are thoroughly mixed. If your mixer is not a heavy-duty mixer, at this point beat the dough for 5 to 10 minutes. With some types of bread you will be able to tell that the gluten is developing because the dough will begin to climb up the beaters. Then knead the rest of the flour in by hand, kneading for about 10 minutes, or until the dough is very smooth and elastic. If you wish to add raisins or nuts to the dough, do it during this hand kneading period.

If your mixer is a heavy-duty mixer, after the liquids are thoroughly mixed in, with the mixer still running, begin adding the rest of the flour around the edges of the bowl ½ cup at a time, mixing well after each addition before adding more flour, until the dough forms a ball and cleans the sides of the bowl. Knead the dough on the speed directed in your mixer manual for 5 to 10 minutes, or until the dough is very elastic and smooth. Turn the dough out onto a floured board and knead it briefly to check the consistency of the dough, kneading in a little more flour if necessary. Raisins or nuts should be added to the dough by hand after the mixer is finished kneading it.

Put the dough into an oiled bowl and turn it once so that the top of the ball is also oiled. Cover it with a towel and let it rise in a warm (85°F to 90°F) place until it has doubled in volume, about 45 minutes to 1 hour, or use the microwave rising method on pages 24 to 25. Punch the dough down and shape it into loaves or rolls as desired. (For loaves, use an 8-inch by 4-inch or 9-inch by 5-inch oiled loaf pan). Allow it to rise until double again. Bake loaves at 350°F to 375°F, usually for 45 minutes to an hour, and rolls at 375°F for 15 to 25 minutes.

Depending on the capacity of your mixer's bowl and the power of its motor, you can double, triple, or quadruple the recipes given for bread machines and make several loaves of bread at once. The following sample recipes are for two loaves of bread each.

Mixer White Bread

4 cups bread flour
3½ teaspoons active dry or quick-rise yeast
2 teaspoons salt
¼ cup Fruit Sweet™ or honey warmed to 120°F
1¾ cups water or milk at about 120°F
2 tablespoons oil
1 tablespoon liquid lecithin or additional oil
2¼ to 2½ cups bread flour

Prepare the dough as in the mixer bread directions on page 47. After the first rise, punch down the dough and shape it into two loaves. Put each loaf into an oiled loaf pan. Let the loaves rise until they have doubled again, about 45 minutes if made with active dry yeast. Bake at 375°F for 40 to 45 minutes. Immediately remove the bread from the pans and cool it on a wire rack. Makes 2 loaves. This recipe may be doubled if your mixer is capable of kneading four loaves of bread. The dough from this recipe can also be used to make rolls or buns (pages 112 to 120), pizza (page 154), breadsticks (page 158), or pretzels (page 160). The nutritional analysis for this bread is about the same as for two large loaves of "White Bread," page 60.

Mixer White Spelt Bread

4 cups white spelt flour
3½ teaspoons active dry or quick-rise yeast
1½ teaspoons salt
⅜ cup apple juice concentrate warmed to 120°F
1¼ cups water at about 120°F
5 teaspoons oil
2 teaspoons liquid lecithin or additional oil
1¾ to 2 cups white spelt flour

Prepare the dough as in the mixer bread directions on page 47. After the first rise, punch down the dough and shape it into two loaves. Put each loaf into an oiled loaf pan. Let the loaves rise until they have doubled again, about 45 minutes if made with active dry yeast. Bake at 375°F for 40 to 45 minutes. Immediately remove the bread from the pans and cool it on a wire rack. Makes 2 loaves. This recipe may be doubled if your mixer is capable of kneading four loaves of bread. The dough from this recipe can also be used to make rolls or buns (pages 112 to 120), pizza (page 155), breadsticks (page 158), or pretzels (page 160). The nutritional analysis for this bread is the same as for two large loaves of "White Spelt Bread," page 61.

Mixer Whole Wheat Bread

4½ cups whole wheat bread flour
2 packages (4½ teaspoons) active dry or quick-rise yeast
2 teaspoons salt
½ cup apple juice concentrate warmed to 120°F
2¼ cups water at about 120°F
2 tablespoons oil
1 tablespoon liquid lecithin or additional oil
3 to 3¼ cups whole wheat bread flour

Prepare the dough as in the mixer bread directions on page 47. After the first rise, punch down the dough and shape it into two loaves. Put each loaf into an oiled loaf pan. Let the loaves rise until they have doubled again, about 45 minutes if made with active dry yeast. Bake at 375°F for 40 to 45 minutes. Immediately remove the bread from the pans and cool it on a wire rack. Makes 2 loaves. This recipe may be doubled if your mixer is capable of kneading four loaves of bread. The dough from this recipe can also be used to make rolls or buns (pages 112 to 120), pizza (page 154), breadsticks (page 158), or pretzels (page 160). The nutritional analysis for this bread is the same as for two large loaves of "100% Whole Wheat Bread," page 74.

Mixer Spelt Bread

4 cups spelt flour
2 packages (4½ teaspoons) active dry or quick-rise yeast
1¼ teaspoons salt
⅓ cup apple juice concentrate warmed to 120°F
1⅔ cup water at about 120°F
2 tablespoons oil
1 tablespoon liquid lecithin or additional oil
2¼ to 2¾ cups spelt flour

Prepare the dough as in the mixer bread directions on page 47. After the first rise, punch down the dough and shape it into two loaves. Put each loaf into an oiled loaf pan. (This bread can be difficult to remove from the pan after baking, especially if you have baked it for the full baking time. If you prefer your bread well browned, also line each pan with oiled waxed or parchment paper). Let the loaves rise until they have doubled again, about 45 minutes if made with active dry yeast. Bake at 375°F for 40 to 45 minutes. Immediately remove the bread from the pans and cool it on a wire rack. Makes 2 loaves. This recipe may be doubled if your mixer is capable of kneading four loaves of bread. The dough from this recipe can also be used to make rolls or buns (pages 112 to 120), pizza (page 154), breadsticks (page 158), or pretzels (page 160). The nutritional analysis for this bread is the same as for two large loaves of "Whole Grain Spelt Bread," page 76.

Mixer Kamut Bread

4 cups kamut flour
2 packages (4½ teaspoons) active dry or quick-rise yeast
1½ teaspoon salt
2½ cups water at about 120°F
½ cup apple or pineapple juice concentrate warmed to 120°F
3 tablespoons oil
2½ to 3 cups kamut flour

Prepare the dough as in the mixer bread directions on page 47 except do not let it rise the first time. After checking its consistency, shape it into two loaves. Put each loaf into an oiled 8-inch by 4-inch loaf pan. Let the loaves rise until they double or reach the top of the pans, about 30 to 50 minutes. Bake at 375°F for 40 to 45 minutes. Immediately remove the bread from the pans and cool it on a wire rack. Makes 2 loaves. This recipe may be doubled if your mixer is capable of kneading four loaves of bread. The dough from this recipe can also be used to make rolls or buns (pages 112 to 120), pizza (page 154), breadsticks (page 158), or pretzels (page 160). The nutritional analysis for this bread is the same as for two small loaves of "Kamut Bread," page 84.

Mixer Brown Bread

4 cups white rye flour

3 packages (6¾ teaspoons) active dry or quick-rise yeast

1 tablespoon salt

2 tablespoons caraway seeds

½ cup carob (optional; if omitted, add an extra ½ cup of white rye flour)

2 cups water at about 120°F

½ cup dark molasses

2 tablespoons oil

3¼ to 3¾ cups white rye flour

Prepare the dough as in the mixer bread directions on page 47. After the first rise, punch down the dough and shape it into two balls. Place them on oiled baking sheets and slash the tops of the loaves. Let them rise until double in volume, about one hour if made with active dry yeast. Bake at 375°F for 35 to 45 minutes. Immediately remove the bread from the baking sheets and cool it on a wire rack. Makes 2 loaves. This recipe may be doubled if your mixer is capable of kneading four loaves of bread. The nutritional analysis for this bread is the same as for two loaves of "Brown Bread," page 79.

MIXER BREADS MADE WITH GLUTEN-FREE AND LOW-GLUTEN FLOURS

Gluten-free and low-gluten breads are much different to make than high-gluten breads. Instead of your mixer developing the gluten, it "develops" the guar gum structure of the bread. Because low-gluten and gluten-free bread dough is much softer, ranging in consistency from a heavy batter to a soft dough, all of the "kneading" can be done by your mixer even if it is not a heavy duty mixer. The beating times are shorter (about 3 minutes) for gluten-free and low-gluten breads than for gluten-containing mixer breads. Also, you beat the dough twice, once initially and once after the first rising period. The method used in the two sample rice bread recipes below can also be used to make barley, oat, amaranth, quinoa, and buckwheat breads and gluten-free rolls or sweet rolls. (See the bread machine recipes for these breads on pages 82, 83, bottom of 84, 85, and top of 86). Use the same amounts of all of the ingredients as in the bread machine recipes. The rising and baking times will vary with the type of bread you make. Just let the bread rise until it barely doubles and bake it until it is brown. DO NOT let these breads over-rise in the pan or they will collapse during baking.

Mixer Rice Bread

2 cups brown rice flour or white rice flour
1/3 cup potato flour
1/3 cup tapioca flour
1 package (2 1/4 teaspoons) active dry or quick-rise yeast
4 teaspoons guar gum
1/8 teaspoon unbuffered vitamin C crystals
1 teaspoon salt
2 tablespoon oil
3 extra-large eggs OR 3/4 cup egg substitute at room temperature
1/4 cup apple juice concentrate at about 115°F
1/2 cup water at about 115°F

Combine the flours, yeast, guar gum, vitamin C crystals, and salt in your mixer bowl and mix for about 30 seconds. Beat the eggs slightly and combine them with the water, juice, and oil in a separate bowl or cup. With the mixer running, add the liquid ingredients to the bowl. When the ingredients are completely combined, beat the dough for three minutes at medium speed. Scrape the dough from the beaters and the sides of the bowl into the bottom of the bowl. Cover the bowl, put it in a warm (85°F to 90°F) place, and let the dough rise for 1 hour. Beat the dough again for three minutes at medium speed. Oil an 8-inch by 4-inch loaf pan and coat the inside of it generously with rice flour. Put the dough in the pan and allow it to rise in a warm place until it doubles, about 30 to 40 minutes for active dry yeast or 20 to 30 minutes for quick-rise yeast. Preheat the oven to 375°F. Bake for 30 to 45 minutes. Makes one loaf. The nutritional analysis of this recipe is the same as for a large loaf of "Gluten-free Rice Potato Bread," page 72.

Mixer Egg-free Rice Bread

2 3/4 cups brown rice flour
3/4 cup tapioca flour
1 package (2 1/4 teaspoons) active dry or quick-rise yeast
1 tablespoon guar gum
1 teaspoon salt
1 1/2 cup warm (110-115°F) water
3 tablespoons honey or Fruit Sweet™
3 tablespoons oil

Combine the flours, yeast, guar gum, and salt in your mixer bowl and mix for about 30 seconds. Combine the water, honey or Fruit Sweet™, and oil in a separate bowl or cup. With the mixer running, add the liquid ingredients to the bowl. When the ingredients are completely combined, beat the dough for three minutes at medium speed. Scrape the dough from the beaters and the sides of the bowl into the bottom of the bowl. Cover the bowl, put it in a warm (85°F to 90°F) place, and let the dough rise for 1 hour. Beat the dough again for three minutes at medium speed. Oil a loaf pan and coat the inside of it generously with rice flour. Put the dough in the pan and allow it to rise in a warm place until it doubles, about 25 to 35 minutes for active dry yeast or 20 to 25 minutes for quick-rise yeast. Preheat the oven to 375°F. Bake for 30 to 45 minutes. Makes one loaf. The nutritional analysis of this recipe is the same as for "Egg-free Brown Rice Bread," page 84.

HAND MIXED QUICK BREADS

Quick breads are very easy to make by hand without any machines, but if you are on a yeast-free diet and eat quick breads exclusively, it is nice to have a bread machine that will do the work for you! To make quick breads by hand, first preheat your oven to 350°F and oil and flour your bread pan. Stir together the flour(s), baking powder, baking soda, salt, and other dry ingredients in a large bowl. Combine the liquid ingredients in another bowl or cup. Stir them into the dry ingredients quickly, until they are just barely mixed together, and put the batter into the prepared pan. Bake at 350°F until the bread is nicely browned and a toothpick inserted in the center comes out dry. This may take from 30 to 70 minutes. When using the bread machine quick bread recipes in this book to make quick breads by hand rather than using a bread machine, there is no need to change the amounts of any of the ingredients. Sample hand-mixed quick bread recipes are given on the next two pages to show just how easy it is to make hand-mixed quick breads.

Hand Mixed Corn Bread

1½ cups all purpose flour
½ cup cornmeal
2½ teaspoons baking powder
½ teaspoon salt
2 tablespoons oil
1 extra large egg OR ¼ cup egg substitute OR ¼ cup water in addition to
    the amount below
¼ cup Fruit Sweet™ or honey
⅜ cup water

Preheat your oven to 350°F. Oil and flour an 8-inch by 4-inch loaf pan. Mix together the flour, cornmeal, baking powder, and salt in a large bowl. Combine the oil, egg, sweetener, and water and quickly stir them into the dry ingredients until they are just mixed. Put the batter into the prepared pan and bake at 350°F for 30 to 40 minutes, or until the bread is golden brown and a toothpick inserted into the center comes out clean. The nutritional analysis for this bread is the same as for "Corn Bread," page 128.

Hand Mixed White Spelt Quick Bread

3 cups white spelt flour
3 teaspoons baking powder
½ teaspoon salt
¼ cup oil
1 cup water

Preheat your oven to 350°F. Oil and flour (with white spelt flour) an 8-inch by 4-inch loaf pan. Mix together the flour, baking powder, and salt in a large bowl. Combine the oil and water and quickly stir them into the dry ingredients until they are just mixed. Put the batter into the prepared pan and bake at 350°F for 60 to 70 minutes, or until the bread is golden brown and a toothpick inserted into the center comes out clean. This bread is fragile, so allow it to cool completely before slicing it. The nutritional analysis for this bread is the same as for "No-Yeast White Spelt Bread," page 124.

Hand Mixed White Rice Quick Bread

1⅓ cups white rice flour

⅓ cup tapioca flour

⅓ cup potato flour

2¾ teaspoons guar gum

2¾ teaspoons baking powder

¾ teaspoon salt

1 tablespoon plus 1 teaspoon oil

2 extra-large eggs, slightly beaten OR ½ cup egg substitute

1⅓ cups water

Preheat your oven to 350°F. Oil and flour (with white rice flour) an 8-inch by 4-inch loaf pan. Mix together the flours, baking powder, guar gum, and salt in a large bowl. Combine the oil, eggs, and water and quickly stir them into the dry ingredients until they are just mixed. Put the batter into the prepared pan and bake at 350°F for 55 to 65 minutes, or until the bread is golden brown and a toothpick inserted into the center comes out clean. The nutritional analysis for this bread is the same as for "No-Yeast Gluten-free Rice Bread," page 128.

Instructions and Recipes for Bread Machine Breads

Each bread machine has a personality of its own (at our house when my children were young they even had names), so the first thing you should do when you get a bread machine is get to know it. Read the instruction booklet and any recipes that come with it. Make a basic bread with a recipe the manufacturer provides. Listen to how the machine sounds as it kneads. Reach into the machine and feel the dough. If the times for each part of the cycle are not given in the instruction book, time the parts of the cycle. Peek into the machine and see how the dough looks at every stage of the cycle.

Getting to know your bread machine is helpful in many ways. When you know how it normally sounds, you will recognize the distressed kneading sound it makes if your dough is too stiff and dry. If you know how long each part of the cycle takes, you will know when the last knead ends and can set your kitchen timer to add raisins or nuts near the end of the kneading time. Touch the dough for a loaf of bread made with the manufacturer's recipe to gain experience in how bread machine dough should feel.

An important skill to develop is the ability to judge the consistency of the dough by looking at it and touching it. For high-gluten doughs, such as wheat and spelt, after several minutes of kneading, the dough should form a smooth, silky ball. It should feel slightly tacky but not sticky when you reach into the machine and touch it. Do not judge a bread dough and begin adding flour or water in the first few minutes of kneading; allow the gluten time to develop. (The exception to this is if the machine sounds like it is really laboring to knead. In this case, add water one tablespoon at a time immediately). After several minutes of kneading, if the dough is too wet or too dry, add either flour (one tablespoon at a time) or water (one teaspoon at a time) until the right consistency is reached, allowing the machine to knead for a minute or two after each addition. Using this method, you can compensate for the inevitable variations in flour quality or moisture content due to weather changes.

Record any changes you make in the recipes and how the bread turns out with your changes. If you live in an exceptionally dry or wet climate you may find that you routinely have to use more water or flour than the recipe calls for.

The consistency of lower-gluten doughs varies from recipe to recipe and is difficult to make generalizations about. Rye dough is very sticky. Some gluten-free doughs may look and feel more like heavy batters than doughs. The first time you make each unusual bread, follow the recipe exactly and observe the consistency of the dough carefully. Measuring accurately and using high quality ingredients should produce a good loaf, but if your bread does not come out well, record that, and make the appropriate changes (see below) the next time, again observing the dough. After making a few loaves of each kind of bread, you will gain enough experience to be able to compensate for any variations in your flour. Using high quality commercial flour the first few times you make these types of bread is highly recommended.

The most common problem you will have making non-wheat bread is that the loaf will collapse during baking. This collapse may be very slight, just resulting in a flat-topped loaf, and may not even need correcting, or the collapse can be profound and the loaf can come out with a sunken top or gooey in the middle. There are several possible causes and solutions for this problem. One possible cause is that the dough may have been too wet. Increase the amount of flour or decrease the amount of water the next time you make the bread. Another cause may be that the second rising time is too long. If you have a programmable machine, decrease the last rising time. To slow the rising, you may also decrease the amount of yeast or slightly increase the amount of salt used. You can also try to increase the structure strength of the bread by increasing the amount of guar gum you use. If you are not allergic to eggs, you can strengthen the bread's structure by replacing part of the water called for with eggs, using one extra large egg instead of ¼ cup of water.

It is very important to measure accurately when using a bread machine. To measure flour, stir it to loosen it, lightly spoon it into your measuring cup, and level it off with a straight-edged knife or spatula. To measure liquids, place the measuring cup on a flat surface, and get down so your eye is at the level of the cup to read it. The bottom of the curve of the liquid (meniscus) should line up with the measurement you want to use. When measuring dry ingredients in a measuring spoon, level them off with a straight-edged knife or spatula. When measuring liquids, make sure they do not round up above the top of the spoon.

All ingredients should be at or slightly above room temperature when they go into the bread machine. Eggs can be warmed up quickly by immersing them in warm tap water for a few minutes. Microwave ovens are great for bringing other cold ingredients up to room temperature; just be careful not to microwave them for so long that they become hot.

Add the ingredients to the pan in the order that the manufacturer of your bread machine recommends. This will usually be from the top of the ingredient list in this book down as you read the recipe. Occasionally I have reversed the order by mistake. When I have added the yeast first to a liquids-first machine, the machine had difficulty mixing the dough, but when I added the liquids first to a yeast-first machine there were no problems. When you are using the delayed cycle timer, it is better to add the liquids first and put the yeast in a small well in the top of the flour to insure that it stays dry even if you use a machine in which you normally add the yeast first. The ingredients are listed in a specific order in each recipe to keep the yeast from coming into contact with the salt, oil, or liquids during any waiting time before the machine mixes the dough.

Most of the time bread machines do not need any attention after you start them and check the dough's consistency, but if you are going to be nearby when they are running, it can be worth your while to peek into them a couple of times during the cycle. If you check the dough's consistency after the first several minutes of mixing, you will know if you forgot to put in a cup of the flour or if the weather has made a little adjustment necessary, and you can correct the problem early to insure a good loaf of bread. If you look into the machine during the rising time, you will be able to puncture the dough with a pin if it is threatening to rise over the edge of the pan. (This should only occur if you are "experimenting"). Also, by checking in the middle of the cycle, you will discover if you have forgotten to add the yeast. (I have done this many times!) Don't despair if you forget the yeast. Just mix it with one to two tablespoons of warm water, remove the dough from the machine, and knead the yeast mixture into the dough. Replace the dough in the pan, restart the cycle, and your bread with be all right.

When you make bread with some of the unusual non-wheat flours, the machine may require some assistance in mixing the batter or dough. This usually involves using a slim rubber spatula to detach the dough from the sides of the pan and possibly pushing the upper central part of the dough to the side so it will be thoroughly mixed in. For some machines, especially those with rectangular pans, you may also need use the rubber spatula to carefully turn the dough over in the pan. Most bread machine instruction booklets caution against inserting any utensils into the machine while it is running, but to make many non-wheat breads, careful assistance with a rubber spatula during mixing is a necessity. Also, for some recipes, it is helpful to spread the dough or batter evenly in the pan after the last kneading before the final rise and bake parts of the cycle.

All of the recipes in this book were baked on a medium crust darkness setting. If your machine has a crust color selection feature, the first time you make each recipe, use the medium setting. Then if you prefer your crust darker or lighter, make a note of it and try a different setting the next time.

The recipes in this book give the amounts of ingredients to use to make 1 pound or 1½ pound loaves. If your machine makes 2 pound loaves, first try making a 1½ pound loaf to see if it almost fills the pan. If it does, a 2 pound loaf will probably be a "lid thumper." If not, you can make a 2 pound loaf by doubling the amounts of the ingredients given for a 1 pound loaf. If the loaf is very large, decrease the yeast by ¼ to ½ teaspoon the next time.

WHAT TO DO IF...

If you find that your bread is not as light and fluffy as you'd like, you may try increasing the amount of the yeast slightly. Some experienced bakers routinely use about 3 teaspoons of yeast for each 1½ pound loaf of bread because they prefer very light bread. This may lead to over-rising and collapse with some non-wheat breads, however.

If you live at a very high altitude (over 7000 feet) and your bread over-proofs and collapses during baking, try decreasing the amount of yeast called for in the recipe by one-fourth to one-third.

If you live in a very humid or very dry climate or if you are baking on an exceptionally dry or rainy day, you may need to compensate for the humidity, or lack of it, when you make bread. Check the dough after several minutes of kneading (see page 56) and add extra water one teaspoon at a time or extra flour one tablespoon at a time if necessary. Record how much extra flour or water you add; you may need to make this change every time if you live in a very dry or humid location.

If you already have a non-programmable machine and want to make breads that require a programmable cycle, you can use the dough cycle of your machine to make the dough and allow it to rise the first time. Then punch or stir down the dough and transfer it to an oiled loaf pan, allow it to rise until barely doubled, and bake it in the oven at 350°F until it is nicely browned. For very dense breads, this may take over an hour.

If your machine does not have a whole grain cycle and your whole grain breads come out very dense, they may benefit from some extra kneading time. Simply stop the machine and start the cycle over again after the first 15 to 20 minutes of kneading and then let the cycle proceed normally.

If your machine has a rectangular pan and you notice that there are floury patches on the corners of the finished loaf of bread, the next time you bake, check the bread after it has kneaded for several minutes. If there is still flour in the corners of the pan, use a rubber spatula to move it so it will be kneaded into the dough. This is especially likely to happen if you machine has only one kneading bar and makes a near normal shaped loaf of bread.

If your bread does not rise at all, think back. Did you remember to put the yeast into the machine? If you discover that you forgot the yeast before the "bake" part of the cycle begins, all is not lost. See page 58 for what to do if you forget the yeast.

If you have other problems, you may wish to call your bread machine manufacturer for advice. Also, Red Star Yeast has a bread machine information line (800-445-4746). Along with answering your questions, they may send you coupons to use the next time you purchase Red Star yeast.

Basic Breads

White Bread

Ingredients:	1½ pound loaf	1 pound loaf
Water or milk	1 cup	⅔ cups
Fruit Sweet™ or honey	2 tablespoons	4 teaspoons
Oil	1 tablespoon	2 teaspoons
Liquid lecithin (or may use additional oil)	½ tablespoon	1 teaspoon
Salt	1 teaspoon	¾ teaspoon
Bread flour	3 cups	2 cups
Active dry yeast*	1¾ teaspoons	1¼ teaspoons

Cycle: Basic yeast bread

*Note: I routinely use SAF™ Red instant yeast and the quick basic cycle on my Zojirushi Home Bakery to make this bread. See page 39 for more information about this.

Nutritional analysis per serving: 82 cal, 2.3 g protein, 15 g carbohydrate, 1.2 g fat, 0 g sat fat, 0 mg cholesterol, 107 mg sodium, 0.05 g fiber
Serving size: approximately 1.2 ounce
Servings per large loaf: 19, per small loaf: 14
Diabetic exchanges: 1 starch/bread per serving

No-Salt-Added White Bread

Ingredients:	1½ pound loaf	1 pound loaf
Water	⅔ cup	⅜ cup + 1 tablespoon
Apple juice concentrate, thawed	3 tablespoons	2 tablespoons
Oil	2 teaspoons	1½ teaspoons
Liquid lecithin (or may use additional oil)	1 teaspoon	1 teaspoon
Bread flour	2⅛ cups + 1 tablespoon	1½ cups +1 tablespoon
Active dry yeast	1¼ teaspoons	¾ teaspoon

Cycle: Basic yeast bread

Nutritional analysis per serving: 79 cal, 2 g protein, 14.3 g carbohydrate, 1 g fat, 0 g sat fat, 0 mg
cholesterol, 1.5 mg sodium, 0.05 g fiber
    Serving size: approximately 1.0 ounce
    Servings per large loaf: 15, **per small loaf:** 10
    Diabetic exchanges: 1 starch/bread per serving

White Spelt Bread

Ingredients:	**1½ pound loaf**	**1 pound loaf**
Water	¾ cup	⅔ cup
Apple juice concentrate, thawed	3 tablespoons	2 tablespoons
Oil	2½ teaspoons	2 teaspoons
Liquid lecithin (or may use additional oil)	1 teaspoon	1 teaspoon
Salt	¾ teaspoon	½ teaspoon
White spelt flour	2⅞ cups	2⅜ cups
Active dry yeast	1¾ teaspoons	1¼ teaspoons

Cycle: Basic yeast bread

Note: I routinely use active dry yeast and the quick basic cycle on my Zojirushi Home
Bakery to make this bread.

Nutritional analysis per serving: 80 cal, 3 g protein, 15 g carbohydrate, 1.2 g fat, 0 g sat fat, 0 mg
cholesterol, 1.5 mg sodium, 0.05 g fiber
    Serving size: approximately 1.0 ounce
    Servings per large loaf: 15, **per small loaf:** 10
    Diabetic exchanges: 1 starch/bread per serving

No-Salt-Added White Spelt Bread

Ingredients: **1½ pound loaf**

Water   ⅔ cup
Apple juice concentrate, thawed   2 tablespoons + 2 teaspoons
Oil   2 teaspoons
Liquid lecithin (or may use additional oil)   1 teaspoon
White spelt flour   2½ cups
Active dry yeast   1½ teaspoons

Cycle for programmable machines: Use the times on the standard cycle except set Rise 1 to the lowest time possible, Rise 2 to 30 minutes, and Bake to 60 minutes.

If you do not have a programmable machine, the quick yeast cycle may be tried for this recipe.

Note: Because the gluten structure of white spelt is fragile without salt, this bread may be somewhat coarse in texture and may collapse slightly during baking.

Nutritional analysis per serving: 83 cal, 3 g protein, 15 g carbohydrate, 1.2 g fat, 0 g sat fat, 0 mg
        cholesterol, 1.7 mg sodium, 0.3 g fiber
   Serving size: approximately 1.0 ounce
   Servings per loaf: 15
   Diabetic exchanges: 1 starch/bread per serving

Italian Bread

Ingredients: **1, 1½, or 2 pound machine**

Water   1¼ cups
Apple juice concentrate, thawed   1½ tablespoons
Salt   1½ teaspoons
Bread flour   3¼ cups
Active dry yeast   2¼ teaspoons

Cycle: Dough cycle. Remove the dough from the machine at the end of the cycle and knead it briefly on an oiled or very lightly floured board. Shape it into a long or round loaf, or divide it into three pieces, roll them into 15-inch ropes, and braid the dough. Place the loaf on a baking sheet that has been oiled and sprinkled with cornmeal or flour. Let it rise in a warm place until double, 30 to 45 minutes. Preheat your oven to 400°F and, if desired, put in a few potatoes to bake along with the bread for added moisture to help the crust become crisp. Spray the bread with water right before baking. Bake for 25 to 40 minutes, spraying it with water twice more after 5 and 10 minutes of baking.

Nutritional analysis per serving: 76 cal, 3 g protein, 15 g carbohydrate, 0.2 g fat, 0 g sat fat, 0 mg cholesterol, 168 mg sodium, 0.06 g fiber
Serving size: approximately 1.3 ounce
Servings per loaf: 18
Diabetic exchanges: 1 starch/bread per serving

Wheat-Free Italian Bread

Ingredients:	**1, 1½, or 2 pound machine**
Water	1¼ cups
Apple juice concentrate, thawed	1½ tablespoons
Salt	1½ teaspoons
White spelt flour	3¾ cups
Active dry yeast	1¼ teaspoons

Cycle: Dough cycle. Remove the dough from the machine at the end of the cycle and knead it briefly on an oiled or very lightly floured board. Shape it into a long or round loaf, or divide it into three pieces, roll them into 15-inch ropes, and braid the dough. Place the loaf on a baking sheet that has been oiled and sprinkled with cornmeal or white spelt flour. Let it rise in a warm place until double, 30 to 45 minutes. Preheat your oven to 400°F and, if desired, put in a few potatoes to bake along with the bread for added moisture to help the crust become crisp. Spray the bread with water right before baking. Bake for 25 to 40 minutes, spraying it with water twice more after 5 and 10 minutes of baking.

Nutritional analysis per serving: 81 cal, 3 g protein, 16 g carbohydrate, 0.4 g fat, 0 g sat fat, 0 mg cholesterol, 151 mg sodium, 0.4 g fiber
Serving size: approximately 1.2 ounce
Servings per loaf: 20
Diabetic exchanges: 1 starch/bread per serving

French Bread

Ingredients: **1, 1½, or 2 pound machine**

Water	1¼ cups
Apple juice concentrate, thawed	1½ tablespoons
Salt	1½ teaspoons
Bread flour	3¼ cups
Active dry yeast	2¼ teaspoons

½ slightly beaten egg white OR "Bread or Bun Wash," page 111.

Cycle: Dough cycle, using the ingredients above the line. Remove the dough from the machine at the end of the cycle and knead it briefly on an oiled or very lightly floured board. Shape it into a long loaf or two very thin long loaves. Put it into oiled French bread or baguette pan or on a baking sheet that has been oiled and sprinkled with cornmeal or flour. Brush with egg white or bread wash, slash the top diagonally, and let it rise in a warm place until double, about 30 to 45 minutes. If desired, brush again right before baking. Preheat your oven to 400°F and, if desired, put in a few potatoes to bake along with the bread for added moisture to help the crust become crisp. Bake for 20 to 40 minutes, or until nicely browned.

Nutritional analysis per serving: 77 cal, 3 g protein, 15 g carbohydrate, 0.2 g fat, 0 g sat fat, 0 mg
      cholesterol, 168 mg sodium, 0.06 g fiber
Serving size: approximately 1.3 ounce
Servings per loaf: 18
Diabetic exchanges: 1 starch/bread per serving

Wheat-Free French Bread

Ingredients: **1, 1½, or 2 pound machine**

Water	1¼ cups
Apple juice concentrate, thawed	1½ tablespoons
Salt	1½ teaspoons
White spelt flour	3¾ cups
Active dry yeast	2¼ teaspoons

½ slightly beaten egg white OR "Bread or Bun Wash," page 111.

Cycle: Dough cycle, using the ingredients above the line. Remove the dough from the machine at the end of the cycle and knead it briefly on an oiled or very lightly floured board. Shape it into a long loaf or two very thin long loaves. Put it into oiled French bread or baguette pan or on a baking sheet that has been oiled and sprinkled with cornmeal or white spelt flour. Brush with egg white or bread wash, slash the top diagonally, and let it rise in a warm place until double, about 30 to 45 minutes. If desired, brush again right before baking. Preheat your oven to 400°F and, if desired, put in a few potatoes to bake along with the bread for added moisture to help the crust become crisp. Bake for 20 to 40 minutes, or until nicely browned.

Nutritional analysis per serving: 82 cal, 3 g protein, 16 g carbohydrate, 0.4 g fat, 0 g sat fat, 0 mg cholesterol, 151 mg sodium, 0.4 g fiber
Serving size: approximately 1.2 ounce
Servings per loaf: 20
Diabetic exchanges: 1 starch/bread per serving

Oat Bran Bread

Ingredients:	**1½ pound loaf**	**1 pound loaf**
Water	1 cup	¾ cup
Apple juice concentrate, thawed	¼ cup	3 tablespoons
Oil	2 teaspoons	1½ teaspoons
Liquid lecithin (or may use additional oil)	1 teaspoon	½ teaspoon
Salt	1 teaspoon	¾ teaspoon
Bread flour	2⅔ cups	2 cups
Oat bran	¾ cup	½ cup + 1 tablespoon
Active dry yeast	1¾ teaspoons	1¼ teaspoons

Cycle: Basic yeast bread

Nutritional analysis per serving: 84 cal, 2.6 g protein, 15 g carbohydrate, 1.4 g fat, 0 g sat fat, 0 mg cholesterol, 113 mg sodium, 0.3 g fiber
Serving size: approximately 1.3 ounce
Servings per large loaf: 18, **per small loaf:** 14
Diabetic exchanges: 1 starch/bread per serving

No-Salt-Added Oat Bran Bread

Ingredients:	1½ pound loaf	1 pound loaf
Water	¾ cup	⅝ cup
Apple juice concentrate, thawed	3 tablespoons	2 tablespoons+ ¾ teaspoon
Oil	2 teaspoons	1 teaspoon
Liquid lecithin (or may use additional oil)	1 teaspoon	1 teaspoon
Bread flour	2 cups	1½ cups
Oat bran	½ cup + 1 tablespoon	⅜ cup + 2 teaspoons
Active dry yeast	1¼ teaspoons	¾ teaspoon

Cycle: Basic yeast bread

Nutritional analysis per serving: 80 cal, 2.5 g protein, 14 g carbohydrate, 1.3 g fat, 0 g sat fat, 0 mg cholesterol, 2.3 mg sodium, 0.8 g fiber
Serving size: approximately 1.2 ounce
Servings per large loaf: 14, **per small loaf:** 11
Diabetic exchanges: 1 starch/bread per serving

Wheat-Free Oat Bran Bread

Ingredients:	1½ pound loaf	1 pound loaf
Water	1 cup	¾ cup + 1 tablespoon
Apple juice concentrate, thawed	¼ cup	3 tablespoons
Oil	1 tablespoon	2 teaspoons
Liquid lecithin (or may use additional oil)	½ tablespoon	1 teaspoon
Salt	¾ teaspoon	½ teaspoon
White spelt flour	3 cups	2⅓ cups
Oat bran	¾ cup	½ cup + 1 tablespoon
Active dry yeast	2¼ teaspoons	1½ teaspoons

Cycle: Basic yeast bread

Nutritional analysis per serving: 85 cal, 3 g protein, 15 g carbohydrate, 1.4 g fat, 0 g sat fat, 0 mg
cholesterol, 77 mg sodium, 0.7 g fiber
  Serving size: approximately 1.2 ounce
  Servings per large loaf: 20, **per small loaf:** 16
  Diabetic exchanges: 1 starch/bread per serving

Oatmeal Bread

Ingredients:	**1½ pound loaf**	**1 pound loaf**
Boiling water	1 cup	¾ cup
Uncooked rolled oats or quick rolled oats	½ cup	⅜ cup
Apple juice concentrate, thawed	¼ cup	3 tablespoons
Oil	1 tablespoon	2 teaspoons
Liquid lecithin (or may use additional oil)	½ tablespoon	1 teaspoon
Salt	1 teaspoon	¾ teaspoon
Bread flour	2⅝ cups	2 cups
Active dry yeast	1¾ teaspoons	1¼ teaspoons

Cycle: Basic yeast bread. About 20 to 30 minutes before beginning this recipe, mix the boiling water and oats and allow them to cool to room temperature or at least to lukewarm. Then add them to the bread machine with the rest of the liquid ingredients.

Nutritional analysis per serving: 79 cal, 2.3 g protein, 14.3 g carbohydrate, 1.4 g fat, 0 g sat fat, 0 mg
cholesterol, 107 mg sodium, 0.3 g fiber
  Serving size: approximately 1.1 ounce
  Servings per large loaf: 19, **per small loaf:** 15
  Diabetic exchanges: 1 starch/bread per serving

Wheat-Free Oatmeal Bread

Ingredients:	1½ pound loaf	1 pound loaf
Boiling water	1 cup	¾ cup
Uncooked rolled oats or quick rolled oats	½ cup	⅜ cup
Apple juice concentrate, thawed	¼ cup	3 tablespoons
Oil	1 tablespoon	2 teaspoons
Liquid lecithin (or may use additional oil)	½ tablespoon	1 teaspoon
Salt	1 teaspoon	¾ teaspoon
White spelt flour	3 cups	2⅓ cups
Active dry yeast	2 teaspoons	1½ teaspoons

Cycle: Basic yeast bread. About 20 to 30 minutes before beginning this recipe, mix the boiling water and oats and allow them to cool to room temperature or at least to lukewarm. Then add them to the bread machine with the rest of the liquid ingredients.

Nutritional analysis per serving: 81 cal, 2.8 g protein, 15 g carbohydrate, 1.4 g fat, 0 g sat fat, 0 mg
    cholesterol, 97 mg sodium, 0.4 g fiber
Serving size: approximately 1.1 ounce
Servings per large loaf: 21, **per small loaf:** 16
Diabetic exchanges: 1 starch/bread per serving

White Corn Bread

Ingredients:	1½ pound loaf	1 pound loaf
Water	⅞ cup	⅔ cup
Apple juice concentrate, thawed	¼ cup	3 tablespoons
Oil	1 tablespoon	2 teaspoons
Liquid lecithin (or more oil)	½ tablespoon	1 teaspoon
Salt	1 teaspoon	¾ teaspoon
Bread flour	2⅞ cups	2⅛ cups
White cornmeal	⅓ cup	¼ cup
Active dry yeast	1¾ teaspoons	1¼ teaspoons

Cycle: Basic yeast bread

Nutritional analysis per serving: 80 cal, 2.1 g protein, 15 g carbohydrate, 1.3 g fat, 0 g sat fat, 0 mg
cholesterol, 107 mg sodium, 0.06 g fiber
    Serving size: approximately 1.2 ounce
    Servings per large loaf: 20, **per small loaf:** 15
    Diabetic exchanges: 1 starch/bread per serving

Wheat-Free White Corn Bread

Ingredients:	1½ pound loaf	1 pound loaf
Water	⅞ cup	⅔ cup
Apple juice concentrate, thawed	¼ cup	3 tablespoons
Oil	1 tablespoon	2 teaspoons
Liquid lecithin (or may use additional oil)	½ tablespoon	1 teaspoon
Salt	1 teaspoon	¾ teaspoon
White spelt flour	3⅛ cup + 1 tablespoon	2⅜ cup
White cornmeal	⅓ cup	¼ cup
Active dry yeast	1¾ teaspoons	1¼ teaspoons

Cycle: Basic yeast bread

Nutritional analysis per serving: 80 cal, 2.5 g protein, 14 g carbohydrate, 1.2 g fat, 0 g sat fat, 0 mg
cholesterol, 101 mg sodium, 0.3 g fiber
    Serving size: approximately 1.0 ounce
    Servings per large loaf: 22, **per small loaf:** 16
    Diabetic exchanges: 1 starch/bread per serving

Potato Bread

Ingredients:	1½ pound loaf	1 pound loaf
Potato (amount in cubes)	1 small (4 ounces) or ¾ cup cubes	1 very small (3 ounces) or ½ cup cubes
Water	¾ cup	½ cup
Additional water to bring mixture volume up to	1¼ cups	⅞ cup
Apple juice concentrate, thawed	¼ cup	3 tablespoons
Oil	1 tablespoon	2 teaspoons
Liquid lecithin (or may use additional oil)	½ tablespoon	1 teaspoon
Salt	1 teaspoon	¾ teaspoon
Bread flour	3¼ cups	2⅓ cups
Active dry yeast	1¾ teaspoons	1¼ teaspoons

Cycle: Basic yeast bread. Peel the potato and cut it into ½-inch cubes. Simmer it in the first amount of water until very tender, about 25 to 30 minutes. Cool to lukewarm. Thoroughly mash the potatoes in the water, adding more water to bring the volume of the mixture up to the amount specified above (1¼ cups for the large loaf, ⅞ cup for the small). Add the mixture and the rest of the ingredients to the machine and start the cycle. Since potatoes vary in moisture content, you should check the consistency of this dough after 5 to 10 minutes of kneading and correct it if necessary. (See page 56).

Nutritional analysis per serving: 81 cal, 2.2 g protein, 15 g carbohydrate, 1.1 g fat, 0 g sat fat, 0 mg cholesterol, 97 mg sodium, 0.1 g fiber
Serving size: approximately 1.3 ounce
Servings per large loaf: 21, **per small loaf:** 14
Diabetic exchanges: 1 starch/bread per serving

Wheat-Free Potato Bread

Ingredients:	1½ pound loaf	1 pound loaf
Potato (amount in cubes)	1 small (4 ounces) or ¾ cup cubes	1 very small (3 ounces) or ½ cup cubes
Water	¾ cup	½ cup
Additional water to bring mixture volume up to	1¼ cups	⅞ cup
Apple juice concentrate, thawed	¼ cup	3 tablespoons
Oil	1 tablespoon	2 teaspoons
Liquid lecithin (or may use additional oil)	½ tablespoon	1 teaspoon
Salt	1 teaspoon	¾ teaspoon
Bread flour	4 cups	2¾ cups
Active dry yeast	2¼ teaspoons	1½ teaspoons

Cycle: Basic yeast bread. Peel the potato and cut it into ½-inch cubes. Simmer it in the first amount of water until very tender, about 25 to 30 minutes. Cool to lukewarm. Thoroughly mash the potatoes in the water, adding more water to bring the volume of the mixture up to the amount specified above (1¼ cups for the large loaf, ⅞ cup for the small). Add the mixture and the rest of the ingredients to the machine and start the cycle. Since potatoes vary in moisture content, you should check the consistency of this dough after 5 to 10 minutes of kneading and correct it if necessary. (See page 56).

Nutritional analysis per serving: 80 cal, 2.7 g protein, 15 g carbohydrate, 1.1 g fat, 0 g sat fat, 0 mg cholesterol, 78 mg sodium, 0.4 g fiber
Serving size: approximately 1.1 ounce
Servings per large loaf: 26, **per small loaf:** 18
Diabetic exchanges: 1 starch/bread per serving

Gluten-Free Rice Potato Bread

Ingredients:	1½ pound loaf	1 pound loaf
Water	½ cup + 1 tablespoon	½ cup
Apple juice concentrate, thawed	¼ cup	3 tablespoons
Oil	2 tablespoons	1½ tablespoons
Eggs (extra large)	3 eggs	2 eggs
OR egg substitute	OR ¾ cup	OR ½ cup
Salt	1 teaspoon	¾ teaspoon
Vitamin C crystals	⅛ teaspoon	Scant ⅛ teaspoon
Guar gum	4 teaspoons	3 teaspoons
Brown rice flour	2 cups	1½ cups
OR white rice flour		
Potato flour	⅓ cup	¼ cup
Tapioca flour	⅓ cup	¼ cup
Active dry yeast	2¼ teaspoons	1½ teaspoons

Cycle: Basic yeast bread

Nutritional analysis per serving if made with eggs: 79 cal, 2.3 g protein, 14 g carbohydrate, 2.2 g fat, 0.2 g sat fat, 43 mg cholesterol, 98 mg sodium, 0.7 g fiber
Nutritional analysis per serving if made with egg substitute: 78 cal, 2.3 g protein, 14 g carbohydrate, 2.5 g fat, 0 g sat fat, 0 mg cholesterol, 99 mg sodium, 0.7 g fiber
Serving size: approximately 1.1 ounce
Servings per large loaf: 24, **per small loaf:** 17
Diabetic exchanges: 1 starch/bread per serving

Whole Grain and Extra Nutrition Breads

Cracked Wheat Bread

Ingredients:	1½ pound loaf	1 pound loaf
Cracked wheat	¼ cup	2 tablespoons
Water	1 cup	½ cup
Water	¾ cup	½ cup + 1 tablespoon
Apple juice concentrate, thawed	3 tablespoons	2½ tablespoons
Oil	2 teaspoons	1½ teaspoons
Liquid lecithin (or may use additional oil)	1 teaspoon	½ teaspoon
Salt	¾ teaspoon	½ teaspoon
Cooked cracked wheat	½ cup	⅜ cup
Bread flour	2⅛ cups	1⅝ cups
Whole wheat bread flour	½ cup	⅜ cup
Active dry yeast	1¾ teaspoons	1¼ teaspoons

Cycle: Basic yeast bread. A few hours before or the night before making this bread, combine the uncooked cracked wheat and first amount of water listed above the line at the top of the recipe in a saucepan, bring to a boil, reduce the heat, and simmer 15 minutes. Drain the cracked wheat thoroughly in a strainer and allow it to cool to lukewarm or room temperature. Measure the amount of cooked cracked wheat specified below the line in the recipe and add it to the machine with the rest of the ingredients.

Nutritional analysis per serving: 78 cal, 2.4 g protein, 15 g carbohydrate, 1 g fat, 0 g sat fat, 0 mg cholesterol, 81 mg sodium, 0.2 g fiber
Serving size: approximately 1.3 ounce
Servings per large loaf: 19, **per small loaf:** 14
Diabetic exchanges: 1 starch/bread per serving

Traditional Whole Wheat Bread

Ingredients:	1½ pound loaf	1 pound loaf
Water	1 cup	¾ cup + 1 tablespoon
Apple juice concentrate, thawed	¼ cup	3 tablespoons
Oil	1½ tablespoons	1 tablespoon
Liquid lecithin (or may use additional oil)	½ tablespoon	½ tablespoon
Salt	1 teaspoon	¾ teaspoon
Bread flour	1¾ cups	1⅜ cups
Whole wheat bread flour	1½ cups	1¼ cups
Vital gluten (optional)	1 tablespoon	2 teaspoons
Active dry yeast	2 teaspoons	1½ teaspoons

Cycle: Basic yeast bread or quick yeast bread. (I routinely use the "quick" whole grain cycle on my Zojirushi Home Bakery to make this bread).

Nutritional analysis per serving: 81 cal, 2.7 g protein, 14.4 g carbohydrate, 1.5 g fat, 0 g sat fat, 0 mg cholesterol, 92 mg sodium, 0.25 g fiber
Serving size: approximately 1.1 ounce
Servings per large loaf: 22, **per small loaf:** 18
Diabetic exchanges: 1 starch/bread per serving

100% Whole Wheat Bread

Ingredients:	1½ pound loaf	1 pound loaf
Water	1¼ cups	1 cup
Apple juice concentrate, thawed	¼ cup	3 tablespoons
Oil	1 tablespoon	1 tablespoon
Liquid lecithin (or may use additional oil)	½ tablespoon	1 teaspoon
Salt	1 teaspoon	¾ teaspoon
Whole wheat bread flour	3¾ cups	3 cups
Vital gluten (optional)	1½ tablespoons	1 tablespoon
Active dry yeast	2¼ teaspoons	1¾ teaspoons

Cycle: Basic yeast bread or whole grain. When making this bread in a 2 pound machine, do not double the 1 pound recipe. Use the 1½ pound recipe.

Nutritional analysis per serving: 81 cal, 2.6 g protein, 15 g carbohydrate, 1.3 g fat, 0 g sat fat, 0 mg cholesterol, 79 mg sodium, 0.8 g fiber
  Serving size: approximately 1.1 ounce
  Servings per large loaf: 26, **per small loaf:** 20
  Diabetic exchanges: 1 starch/bread per serving

White Wheat Bread

If you or members of your family are not real whole wheat fans, this may be the bread for you. It is lighter in color and flavor than 100% whole wheat bread but still has all the nutritional benefits of being made with 100% whole wheat flour. White whole wheat flour can be purchased from the King Arthur Flour Company. (See "Sources," page 211).

Ingredients:	1½ pound loaf	1 pound loaf
Water	1¼ cups	1 cup
Apple juice concentrate, thawed	¼ cup	3 tablespoons
Oil	1 tablespoon	1 tablespoon
Liquid lecithin (or may use additional oil)	½ tablespoon	1 teaspoon
Salt	1 teaspoon	¾ teaspoon
White whole wheat flour	3¾ cups	3 cups
Vital gluten (optional)	1½ tablespoons	1 tablespoon
Active dry yeast	2¼ teaspoons	1¾ teaspoons

Cycle: Basic yeast bread or whole grain. When making this bread in a 2 pound machine, do not double the 1 pound recipe. Use the 1½ pound recipe.

Nutritional analysis per serving: 81 cal, 2.6 g protein, 15 g carbohydrate, 1.3 g fat, 0 g sat fat, 0 mg cholesterol, 79 mg sodium, 0.8 g fiber
  Serving size: approximately 1.1 ounce
  Servings per large loaf: 26, **per small loaf:** 20
  Diabetic exchanges: 1 starch/bread per serving

Whole Grain Spelt Bread

Ingredients:	1½ pound loaf	1 pound loaf
Water	1 cup	¾ cup
Apple juice concentrate, thawed	¼ cup	3 tablespoons
Oil	1 tablespoon	2 teaspoons
Liquid lecithin (or may use additional oil)	½ tablespoon	1 teaspoon
Salt	¾ teaspoon	½ teaspoon
Whole spelt flour	3⅓ cups	2½ cups
Active dry yeast	2¼ teaspoons	1½ teaspoons

Cycle: Basic yeast bread

Nutritional analysis per serving: 79 cal, 2.5 g protein, 14 g carbohydrate, 1.4 g fat, 0 g sat fat, 0 mg cholesterol, 71 mg sodium, 1.2 g fiber
Serving size: approximately 1.0 ounce
Servings per large loaf: 22, **per small loaf:** 16
Diabetic exchanges: 1 starch/bread per serving

Cracked Spelt Bread

Ingredients:	1½ pound loaf
Cracked spelt*	¼ cup
Water	1 cup
Water	¾ cup
Apple juice concentrate, thawed	¼ cup
Oil	1 tablespoon
Liquid lecithin (or use additional oil)	½ tablespoon
Salt	¾ teaspoon
Cooked cracked spelt	½ cup
Whole spelt flour	½ cup
White spelt flour	2¼ cups
Active dry yeast	2 teaspoons

Cycle for programmable machine: Use the times on the standard cycle except set Rise 1 to the lowest time possible, Rise 2 to 35 minutes, and Bake to 50 minutes

Note: If you cannot find cracked spelt, process some whole spelt in a food processor or blender until it is in chunks the size of half of a spelt grain or smaller. A few hours or the night before you plan to make this bread, cook the cracked spelt for 30 minutes in the first amount of water listed above the line at the top of the recipe and thoroughly drain and cool it as described in the "Cracked Wheat Bread" recipe on page 73. Measure ½ cup of cooked cracked spelt into the bread machine pan with the rest of the ingredients.

Nutritional analysis per serving: 79 cal, 2.7 g protein, 15 g carbohydrate, 1.4 g fat, 0 g sat fat, 0 mg cholesterol, 77 mg sodium, 0.9 g fiber
Serving size: approximately 1.1 ounce
Servings per loaf: 20
Diabetic exchanges: 1 starch/bread per serving

Light Rye Bread

Ingredients:	1½ pound loaf	1 pound loaf
Water	1⅛ cups	⅞ cup
Apple juice concentrate, thawed	¼ cup	3 tablespoons
Oil	1 tablespoon	2 teaspoons
Liquid lecithin (or may use additional oil)	½ tablespoon	1 teaspoon
Salt	1 teaspoon	¾ teaspoon
Caraway seed	1 tablespoon	2¼ teaspoons
Bread flour	2⅝ cups	2 cups
Rye flour	1 cup	¾ cup
Active dry yeast	2 teaspoons	1½ teaspoons

Cycle: Basic yeast bread

Nutritional analysis per serving: 82 cal, 2.3 g protein, 15 g carbohydrate, 1.1 g fat, 0 g sat fat, 0 mg cholesterol, 92 mg sodium, 0.8 g fiber
Serving size: approximately 1.0 ounce
Servings per large loaf: 22, **per small loaf:** 17
Diabetic exchanges: 1 starch/bread per serving

Wheat-Free Light Rye Bread

Ingredients:	1½ pound loaf	1 pound loaf
Water	1 cup	¾ cup
Apple juice concentrate, thawed	¼ cup	3 tablespoons
Oil	1 tablespoon	2 teaspoons
Liquid lecithin (or more oil)	½ tablespoon	1 teaspoon
Salt	1 teaspoon	¾ teaspoon
Caraway seed	1 tablespoon	2¼ teaspoons
White spelt flour	3 cups	2¼ cups
Rye flour	1 cup	¾ cup
Active dry yeast	2 teaspoons	1½ teaspoons

Cycle: Basic yeast bread

Nutritional analysis per serving: 83 cal, 2.7g protein, 15 g carbohydrate, 1.3 g fat, 0 g sat fat, 0 mg
   cholesterol, 85 mg sodium, 0.9 g fiber
   Serving size: approximately 1.0 ounce
   Servings per large loaf: 24, **per small loaf:** 19
   Diabetic exchanges: 1 starch/bread per serving

Whole Rye Bread

Ingredients:	1½ pound loaf	1 pound loaf
Water	⅓ cup	¼ cup
White grape juice	1 cup	⅔ cup
Oil	1½ tablespoons	1 tablespoon
Liquid lecithin (or may use additional oil)	½ tablespoon	½ tablespoon
Salt	1½ teaspoons	1 teaspoon
Unbuffered vitamin C crystals	⅛ teaspoon	Scant ⅛ teaspoon
Rye flour	2½ cups	1⅔ cups
Tapioca flour	¾ cup	½ cup
Guar gum	4 teaspoons	3 teaspoons
Active dry yeast	2¼ teaspoons	1½ teaspoons

Cycle: Basic yeast bread. With some machines, you will have to assist the mixing and kneading of this dough with a spatula as described on page 58. For all machines, spread the dough evenly in the pan as soon as the last kneading time is finished. This bread is very dense.

Nutritional analysis per serving: 81 cal, 1.7 g protein, 15 g carbohydrate, 1.4 g fat, 0 g sat fat, 0 mg
        cholesterol, 137 mg sodium, 1.8 g fiber
    Serving size: approximately 1.1 ounce
    Servings per large loaf: 22, **per small loaf:** 15
    Diabetic exchanges: 1 starch/bread per serving

Brown Bread

Ingredients:	**1½ pound loaf**
Water	1 cup
Dark molasses	¼ cup
Oil	1 tablespoon
Liquid lecithin (or may use additional oil)	1 teaspoon
Salt	1½ teaspoons
Caraway seed*	1 tablespoon
White rye flour**	3¼ cups
Carob powder	¼ cup
Active dry yeast	3½ teaspoons

Cycle: Dough cycle. *Omit caraway seed if you are using this bread for a low fiber diet. This dough is very sticky, so you may need to assist the kneading with a spatula. After the cycle finishes, knead the dough briefly on a board that has been lightly floured with white rye flour. Form it into a ball and place it on an oiled baking sheet. Slash the top of the loaf with a sharp knife and let it rise until double, 1 to 1½ hours. Bake at 375°F for 35 to 45 minutes, or until it has browned slightly and sounds hollow when tapped.

Notes: *Omit caraway seed for a low fiber diet. **White rye flour may be purchased from the King Arthur Flour Baker's Catalogue. See "Sources," page 211.

Nutritional analysis per serving: 81 cal, 2.4 g protein, 16 g carbohydrate, 1 g fat, 0 g sat fat, 0 mg
        cholesterol, 124 mg sodium, 0.3 g fiber
    Serving size: approximately 1.0 ounce
    Servings per loaf: 25
    Diabetic exchanges: 1 starch/bread per serving

Pumpernickel Bread

Ingredients:	1½ pound loaf	1 pound loaf
Water	¾ cup + 1 tablespoon	⅔ cup + 1 tablespoon
Dark molasses	¼ cup	3 tablespoons
Oil	1 tablespoon	2½ teaspoons
Salt	1½ teaspoons	1¼ teaspoons
Caraway seed	1 tablespoon	2½ teaspoons
Unbuffered vitamin C crystals	⅛ teaspoon	Scant ⅛ teaspoon
Bread flour	1½ cups	1¼ cups
Rye flour	1¼ cups	1 cup
Carob powder	¼ cup	3 tbsp. + 1 tsp.
Active dry yeast	3 teaspoons	2¼ teaspoons

Cycle: Basic yeast bread. This dough is very sticky. Spread it evenly in the pan as soon as the last kneading time is finished.

Nutritional analysis per serving: 79 cal, 3.1 g protein, 15 g carbohydrate, 1 g fat, 0 g sat fat, 0 mg cholesterol, 155 mg sodium, 1.0 g fiber
Serving size: approximately 1.1 ounce
Servings per large loaf: 20, **per small loaf:** 16
Diabetic exchanges: 1 starch/bread per serving

All-Rye Pumpernickel Bread

Ingredients:	1½ pound loaf	1 pound loaf
Water	1 cup	¾ cup
Dark molasses	¼ cup	3 tablespoons
Oil	1 tablespoon	2½ teaspoons
Salt	1½ teaspoons	1 teaspoon
Caraway seed	1 tablespoon	2½ teaspoons
Unbuffered vitamin C crystals	⅛ teaspoon	Scant ⅛ teaspoon
White rye flour*	2¼ cups	1⅔ cups + 1 tablespoon
Rye flour	1 cup	¾ cup
Carob powder	¼ cup	3 tablespoons
Active dry yeast	3½ teaspoons	2½ teaspoons

Cycle: Basic yeast bread. Reserve about 1 cup of the white rye flour when you measure the ingredients into the machine and add it ¼ cup at a time during the initial kneading period. This dough is very sticky. Spread it evenly in the pan as soon as the last kneading time is finished.

*Note: White rye flour may be purchased from the King Arthur Flour Baker's Catalogue. See "Sources," page 211.

Nutritional analysis per serving: 83 cal, 2.4 g protein, 18 g carbohydrate, 1 g fat, 0 g sat fat, 0 mg cholesterol, 129 mg sodium, 1.0 g fiber
    Serving size: approximately 1.0 ounce
    Servings per large loaf: 24, **per small loaf:** 18
    Diabetic exchanges: 1 starch/bread per serving

White Rye Bread

Ingredients:	1½ pound loaf	1 pound loaf
Water	⅓ cup	¼ cup
White grape juice	1 cup	¾ cup
Oil	2 tablespoons	1 tablespoon
Liquid lecithin (or more oil)	1 tablespoon	2 teaspoons
Salt	1 teaspoon	¾ teaspoon
White rye flour*	3⅞ cups	2⅞ cups
Active dry yeast	2¼ teaspoons	1¾ teaspoons

Cycle: Basic yeast bread. White rye dough is very sticky and may stick to the side of the pan during mixing. In some machines, you may have to use a spatula to turn the dough over and assist in the kneading, especially as the kneading time progresses. Spread the dough evenly in the pan as soon as the last kneading time is finished.

*Note: White rye flour may be purchased from the King Arthur Flour Baker's Catalogue. See "Sources," page 211.

Nutritional analysis per serving: 82 cal, 2.1 g protein, 15 g carbohydrate, 1.7 g fat, 0 g sat fat, 0 mg cholesterol, 72 mg sodium, 0.3 g fiber
    Serving size: approximately 0.9 ounce
    Servings per large loaf: 28, **per small loaf:** 21
    Diabetic exchanges: 1 starch/bread per serving

Amaranth Bread

Ingredients: **1½ pound loaf**

Water	1⅛ cups
Fruit Sweet™ or honey	3 tablespoons
Oil	2 tablespoons
Liquid lecithin (or use additional oil)	1 tablespoon
Salt	1 teaspoon
Guar gum	4 teaspoons
Amaranth flour*	2½ cups
Arrowroot	¾ cup
Active dry yeast	2¼ teaspoons

Cycle for programmable machines: Use the times on the standard cycle except set Rise 1 to the lowest time possible, Rise 2 to 30 minutes, and Bake to 50 minutes. With some machines you may need to *reserve 1 cup of the amaranth flour to add ¼ cup at a time during the initial kneading and assist the kneading with a spatula. Spread the dough evenly in the pan after the last kneading period.

Nutritional analysis per serving: 81 cal, 1.8 g protein, 13 g carbohydrate, 2.7 g fat, 0 g sat fat, 0 mg cholesterol, 92 mg sodium, 0.4 g fiber
Serving size: approximately 1.4 ounce
Servings per loaf: 22
Diabetic exchanges: 1 starch/bread per serving

Buckwheat Bread

Ingredients: **1½ pound loaf**

Water	1¼ cups
Apple or pineapple juice concentrate, thawed	¼ cup
Oil	3 tablespoons
Salt	1 teaspoon
Guar gum	1 tablespoon
Buckwheat flour*	2 cups
Arrowroot or tapioca flour	1¼ cups
Active dry yeast	2¼ teaspoons

Cycle for programmable machines: Use the times on the standard cycle except set Rise 1 to the lowest time possible, Rise 2 to 30 minutes, and Bake to 55 minutes. With some machines you may need to *reserve 1 cup of the buckwheat flour to add ¼ cup at a time during the initial kneading and assist the kneading with a spatula.

Nutritional analysis per serving: 80 cal, 1.6 g protein, 14 g carbohydrate, 2 g fat, 0 g sat fat, 0 mg cholesterol, 92 mg sodium, 0.1 g fiber
Serving size: approximately 1.2 ounce
Servings per loaf: 22
Diabetic exchanges: 1 starch/bread per serving

Quinoa Bread

Ingredients:	**1½ pound loaf**
Water	1 cup
Apple juice concentrate, thawed	⅓ cup
Oil	2 tablespoons
Liquid lecithin (or may use additional oil)	1 tablespoon
Salt	¾ teaspoon
Cinnamon	1 teaspoon
Guar gum	4 teaspoons
Quinoa flour*	2½ cups
Tapioca flour	¾ cup
Active dry yeast	2¼ teaspoons
Raisins (optional)	½ cup

Cycle for programmable machines: Use the times on the standard cycle except set Rise 1 to the lowest time possible, Rise 2 to 40 to 60 minutes, and Bake to 50 minutes. With some machines you may need to *reserve 1 cup of the quinoa flour to add ¼ cup at a time during the initial kneading and assist the kneading with a spatula. Add the raisins 5 to 10 minutes before the end of the last kneading time.

Nutritional analysis per serving: 120 cal, 2.2 g protein, 21 g carbohydrate, 3.3 g fat, 0 g sat fat, 0 mg cholesterol, 96 mg sodium, 0.8 g fiber
Serving size: approximately 1.6 ounce
Servings per loaf: 16
Diabetic exchanges: 1½ starch/bread per serving

Kamut Bread

Ingredients:	1½ pound loaf	1 pound loaf
Water	1⅜ cups	1¼ cups
Apple juice concentrate, thawed	¼ cup	3 tablespoons
Oil	2 tablespoons	1½ tablespoons
Liquid lecithin (or may use additional oil)	1 tablespoon	½ tablespoon
Salt	1 teaspoon	¾ teaspoon
Kamut flour	4 cups	3¼ cups
Active dry yeast	2¾ teaspoons	2¼ teaspoons

Cycle: Basic yeast bread. When making this bread in a 2 pound machine, do not double the 1 pound recipe. Use the 1½ pound recipe.

Nutritional analysis per serving: 82 cal, 1.1 g protein, 15 g carbohydrate, 1.5 g fat, 0 g sat fat, 0 mg cholesterol, 68 mg sodium, 2.3 g fiber
Serving size: approximately 1.3 ounce
Servings per large loaf: 29, **per small loaf:** 22
Diabetic exchanges: 1 starch/bread per serving

No-Egg Brown Rice Bread

Ingredients:	1½ pound loaf
Water	1½ cups
Fruit Sweet™ or honey	3 tablespoons
Oil	2 tablespoons
Liquid lecithin (or use additional oil)	1 tablespoon
Salt	1 teaspoon
Guar gum	1 tablespoon
Brown rice flour*	2¾ cups
Tapioca flour	¾ cup
Active dry yeast	2¼ teaspoons

Cycle for programmable machines: Use the times on the standard cycle except set Rise 1 to the lowest time possible, Rise 2 to 30** minutes, and Bake to 50 minutes. With some machines you may need to *reserve 1 cup of the rice flour to add ¼ cup at a time during the initial kneading and assist the kneading with a spatula.

Note**Rise 2 should last just until the dough has barely doubled and should end before the top of the dough begins to collapse. The first time you make this bread note if this point is reached before 30 minutes; if it is, use a shorter Rise 2 the next time you make the bread.

Nutritional analysis per serving: 83 cal, 1.4 g protein, 15 g carbohydrate, 2 g fat, 0 g sat fat, 0 mg cholesterol, 77 mg sodium, 1.0 g fiber
Serving size: approximately 1.2 ounce
Servings per loaf: 26
Diabetic exchanges: 1 starch/bread per serving

Barley Bread

Ingredients: **1½ pound loaf**

Water	2 cups
Fruit Sweet™ or honey	2 tablespoons
Oil	1½ tablespoons
Liquid lecithin (or use additional oil)	½ tablespoon
Salt	1 teaspoon
Guar gum	3 teaspoons
Barley flour*	3⅓ cups
Active dry yeast	2¼ teaspoons

Cycle for programmable machines: Use the times on the standard cycle except set Rise 1 to the lowest time possible, Rise 2 to 30 minutes, and Bake to 60 minutes. With some machines you may need to *reserve 1 cup of the barley flour to add ¼ cup at a time during the initial kneading and assist the kneading with a spatula.

Nutritional analysis per serving: 81cal, 1.6 g protein, 16 g carbohydrate, 1.4 g fat, 0 g sat fat, 0 mg cholesterol, 91 mg sodium, 0.2 g fiber
Serving size: approximately 1.3 ounce
Servings per loaf: 22
Diabetic exchanges: 1 starch/bread per serving

Oat Bread

Ingredients: **1½ pound loaf**

Water	1½ cups
Oil	2 tablespoons
Liquid lecithin (or may use additional oil)	1 tablespoon
Salt	½ teaspoon
Guar gum	1 tablespoon
Date sugar	½ cup
Oat flour*	2½ cups
Arrowroot	½ cup
Active dry yeast	2¼ teaspoons

Cycle for programmable machines: Use the times on the standard cycle except set Rise 1 to the lowest time possible, Rise 2 to 30 minutes, and Bake to 50 minutes. With some machines you may need to *reserve 1 cup of the oat flour to add ¼ cup at a time during the initial kneading and assist the kneading with a spatula.

Nutritional analysis per serving: 82 cal, 1.8 g protein, 13 g carbohydrate, 2.4 g fat, 0 g sat fat, 0 mg cholesterol, 42 mg sodium, 1.6 g fiber
Serving size: approximately 1.0 ounce
Servings per loaf: 24
Diabetic exchanges: 1 starch/bread per serving

Wheat Germ Bread

Ingredients:	**1½ pound loaf**	**1 pound loaf**
Water	1⅛ cups	¾ cup
Apple juice concentrate, thawed	⅜ cup	¼ cup
Oil	1½ tablespoons	2 teaspoons
Liquid lecithin (or more oil)	½ tablespoon	1 teaspoon
Salt	1 teaspoon	¾ teaspoon
Bread flour	3 cups	2 cups
Whole wheat bread flour	¾ cup	½ cup
Wheat germ	⅜ cup	¼ cup
Active dry yeast	2½ teaspoons	1¾ teaspoons

Cycle: Basic yeast bread

Nutritional analysis per serving: 81 cal, 2.4 g protein, 12 g carbohydrate, 1.4 g fat, 0 g sat fat, 0 mg
   cholesterol, 76 mg sodium, 0.2 g fiber
   Serving size: approximately 1.1 ounce
   Servings per large loaf: 27, **per small loaf:** 18
   Diabetic exchanges: 1 starch/bread per serving

Multi-Grain Bread

Ingredients:	1½ pound loaf	1 pound loaf
Water	1 cup	⅔ cup
Apple juice concentrate, thawed	¼ cup	3 tablespoons
Oil	1 tablespoon	2 teaspoons
Liquid lecithin (or may use additional oil)	½ tablespoon	1 teaspoon
Salt	1 teaspoon	¾ teaspoon
Bread flour	2 cups	1⅓ cups
Whole wheat bread flour	½ cup	⅓ cup
Rye flour	¼ cup	2 tbsp. + 2 tsp.
Cornmeal	¼ cup	2 tbsp. + 2 tsp.
Cooked rice, any kind	¼ cup	2 tbsp. + 2 tsp.
Rolled oats, uncooked	¼ cup	2 tbsp. + 2 tsp.
Sunflower seeds	2 tablespoons	1 tbsp. + 1 tsp.
Sesame seeds	2 tablespoons	1 tbsp. + 1 tsp.
Active dry yeast	2¼ teaspoons	1½ teaspoons

Cycle: Basic yeast bread

Nutritional analysis per serving: 82 cal, 2.4 g protein, 14 g carbohydrate, 2 g fat, 0 g sat fat, 0 mg
   cholesterol, 88 mg sodium, 0.5 g fiber
   Serving size: approximately 1.1 ounce
   Servings per large loaf: 23, **per small loaf:** 16
   Diabetic exchanges: 1 starch/bread per serving

Three Seed Bread

Ingredients:	1½ pound loaf	1 pound loaf
Water	1 cup	¾ cup
Apple juice concentrate, thawed	¼ cup	3 tablespoons
Oil	1½ tablespoons	1 tablespoon
Liquid lecithin (or may use additional oil)	½ tablespoon	1 teaspoon
Salt	1 teaspoon	¾ teaspoon
Bread flour	2 cups	1½ cups
Whole wheat bread flour	1 cup	¾ cup
Poppy seeds	2 tablespoons	1½ tablespoons
Sesame seeds	2 tablespoons	1½ tablespoons
Sunflower seeds	3 tablespoons	2 tablespoons
Active dry yeast	2 teaspoons	1½ teaspoons

Cycle: Basic yeast bread

Nutritional analysis per serving: 80 cal, 2.3 g protein, 12 g carbohydrate, 2.4 g fat, 0 g sat fat, 0 mg cholesterol, 85 mg sodium, 0.4 g fiber
Serving size: approximately 1.0 ounce
Servings per large loaf: 24, **per small loaf:** 18
Diabetic exchanges: 1 starch/bread per serving

Bread of Gold

Ingredients:	1½ pound loaf	1 pound loaf
Water	1 cup	⅔ cup
Apple juice concentrate, thawed	¼ cup	2½ tablespoons
Oil	1½ tablespoons	1 tablespoon
Liquid lecithin (or may use additional oil)	½ tablespoon	1 teaspoon
Salt	1 teaspoon	¾ teaspoon
Bread flour	1¾ cups	1⅛ cups + 1 tablespoon
Kamut flour	1½ cups	1 cup
Active dry yeast	2¼ teaspoons	1½ teaspoons

Cycle: Basic yeast bread

Nutritional analysis per serving: 79 cal, 2.1 g protein, 14.3 g carbohydrate, 1.4 g fat, 0 g sat fat, 0 mg
  cholesterol, 92 mg sodium, 1.1 g fiber
  Serving size: approximately 1.1 ounce
  Servings per large loaf: 22, **per small loaf:** 15
  Diabetic exchanges: 1 starch/bread per serving

Pumpkin Bread

Ingredients:	**1 or 1½ pound loaf**
Water	⅔ cup
Canned pumpkin	⅓ cup
Oil	1 tablespoon
Salt	¾ teaspoon
Cinnamon	½ teaspoon
Allspice	⅛ teaspoon
Nutmeg	⅛ teaspoon
Cloves	⅛ teaspoon
Ginger	⅛ teaspoon
Bread flour	2⅛ cups
Date sugar	¼ cup
Active dry yeast	1½ teaspoons
Raisins	⅓ cup

Cycle: Raisin bread cycle or basic yeast cycle. Add all of the ingredients except the raisins to the machine and start the cycle. If you are using the basic yeast cycle and it has no signal for when to add raisins, set your kitchen timer to remind you to add the raisins 5 to 10 minutes before the last kneading period is finished. This dough seems to liquefy as the cycle progresses, so you may want to scrape down the sides of the pan after the last kneading time.

Nutritional analysis per serving: 82 cal, 2.1 g protein, 16 g carbohydrate, 1.1 g fat, 0 g sat fat, 0 mg
  cholesterol, 95 mg sodium, 0.6 g fiber
  Serving size: approximately 1.1 ounce
  Servings per loaf: 16
  Diabetic exchanges: 1 starch/bread per serving

Wheat-Free Bread of Gold

Ingredients:	1½ pound loaf	1 pound loaf
Water	1 cup	⅔ cup
Apple juice concentrate, thawed	¼ cup	2½ tablespoons
Oil	1½ tablespoons	1 tablespoon
Liquid lecithin (or may use additional oil)	½ tablespoon	1 teaspoon
Salt	1 teaspoon	¾ teaspoon
White spelt flour	1¾ cups	1⅜ cups + 1 tablespoon
Kamut flour	2⅛ cups	1⅜ cup
Active dry yeast	2¼ teaspoons	1½ teaspoons

Cycle: Basic yeast bread

Nutritional analysis per serving: 80 cal, 2.4 g protein, 15 g carbohydrate, 1.4 g fat, 0 g sat fat, 0 mg cholesterol, 85 mg sodium, 1.2 g fiber
Serving size: approximately 1.0 ounce
Servings per large loaf: 24, **per small loaf:** 16
Diabetic exchanges: 1 starch/bread per serving

Protein Bread

This bread is unusual, but tasty, and may be useful to those on low carbohydrate or hypoglycemic diets.

Ingredients:	1½ pound loaf	1 pound loaf
Water	1 cup	⅔ cup
Apple juice concentrate, thawed	¼ cup	2 tbsp. + 2 tsp.
Oil	1 tablespoon	2 teaspoons
Salt	1 teaspoon	¾ teaspoon
Gluten flour	1 cup	⅔ cup
Soy flour	1 cup	⅔ cup
Wheat germ	¾ cup	½ cup
Active dry yeast	1½ teaspoons	1 teaspoon

Cycle: Basic yeast bread

Nutritional analysis per serving: 80 cal, 8.3 g protein, 7 g carbohydrate, 2.2 g fat, 0 g sat fat, 0 mg
cholesterol, 117 mg sodium, 0.3 g fiber
Serving size: approximately 1.0 ounce
Servings per large loaf: 18, **per small loaf:** 12
Diabetic exchanges: ½ starch/bread + ½ lean meat per serving

Wheat-Free Pumpkin Bread

Ingredients:	**1 or 1½ pound loaf**
Water	⅔ cup
Canned pumpkin	⅓ cup
Oil	1 tablespoon
Salt	¾ teaspoon
Cinnamon	½ teaspoon
Allspice	⅛ teaspoon
Nutmeg	⅛ teaspoon
Cloves	⅛ teaspoon
Ginger	⅛ teaspoon
White spelt flour	2⅝ cups
Date sugar	¼ cup
Active dry yeast	1½ teaspoons
Raisins	⅓ cup

Cycle for programmable machines: Use the times on the standard cycle except set Rise 1 to the lowest time possible, Rise 2 to 35 minutes, and Bake to 50 minutes. Add all of the ingredients except the raisins to the machine and start the cycle. If you are using the basic yeast cycle and it has no signal for when to add raisins, set your kitchen timer to remind you to add the raisins 5 to 10 minutes before the last kneading period is finished. This dough seems to liquefy as the cycle progresses, so you may want to scrape down the sides of the pan after the last kneading time.

Nutritional analysis per serving: 81 cal, 2.5 g protein, 16 g carbohydrate, 1.0 g fat, 0 g sat fat, 0 mg
cholesterol, 80 mg sodium, 0.7 g fiber
Serving size: approximately 1.0 ounce
Servings per loaf: 19
Diabetic exchanges: 1 starch/bread per serving

Corny Bread

Ingredients:	1½ pound loaf	1 pound loaf
Water	⅞ cup	⅔ cup
Apple juice concentrate, thawed	¼ cup	3 tablespoons
Oil	1 tablespoon	2 teaspoons
Liquid lecithin (or may use additional oil)	½ tablespoon	1 teaspoon
Salt	1 teaspoon	¾ teaspoon
Bread flour	2¾ cups	2 cups + 1 tablespoon
Cornmeal (yellow)	⅓ cup	¼ cup
Active dry yeast	1¾ teaspoons	1¼ teaspoons

Cycle: Basic yeast bread

Nutritional analysis per serving: 81 cal, 2.2 g protein, 15 g carbohydrate, 1.3 g fat, 0 g sat fat, 0 mg cholesterol, 107 mg sodium, 0.06 g fiber
Serving size: approximately 1.2 ounce
Servings per large loaf: 19, **per small loaf:** 14
Diabetic exchanges: 1 starch/bread per serving

Wheat-Free Corny Bread

Ingredients:	1½ pound loaf	1 pound loaf
Water	⅞ cup	⅔ cup
Apple juice concentrate, thawed	¼ cup	3 tablespoons
Oil	1 tablespoon	2 teaspoons
Liquid lecithin (or may use additional oil)	½ tablespoon	1 teaspoon
Salt	1 teaspoon	¾ teaspoon
White spelt flour	3 cups	2¼ cups
Cornmeal (yellow)	⅓ cup	¼ cup
Active dry yeast	1¾ teaspoons	1¼ teaspoons

Cycle: Basic yeast bread

Nutritional analysis per serving: 84 cal, 2.7 g protein, 14 g carbohydrate, 1.3 g fat, 0 g sat fat, 0 mg
cholesterol, 101 mg sodium, 0.3 g fiber
Serving size: approximately 1.1 ounce
Servings per large loaf: 20, **per small loaf:** 15
Diabetic exchanges: 1 starch/bread per serving

Gluten-Free Corny Bread

Ingredients:	1½ pound loaf	1 pound loaf
Water	½ cup	⅓ cup
Apple juice concentrate, thawed	¼ cup	3 tablespoons
Oil	2 tablespoons	1 tablespoon + 1 teaspoon
Eggs (extra large) OR egg substitute	3 eggs or ¾ cup	2 eggs or ½ cup
Salt	1 teaspoon	¾ teaspoon
Vitamin C crystals	⅛ teaspoon	Scant ⅛ teaspoon
Guar gum	4 teaspoons	3 teaspoons
Brown rice flour	1⅔ cups	1⅛ cups
Cornmeal (yellow)	⅓ cup	¼ cup
Potato flour	⅓ cup	¼ cup
Tapioca flour	⅓ cup	¼ cup
Active dry yeast	2¼ teaspoons	1½ teaspoons

Cycle: Basic yeast bread

Nutritional analysis per serving if made with eggs: 82 cal, 2.9 g protein, 17 g carbohydrate, 2.9 g fat,
0.3 g sat fat, 57 mg cholesterol, 98 mg sodium, 0.8 g fiber
Nutritional analysis per serving if made with egg substitute: 82 cal, 2.9 g protein, 17 g carbohydrate,
3.2 g fat, 0 g sat fat, 0 mg cholesterol, 127 mg sodium, 0.8 g fiber
Serving size: approximately 1.3 ounce
Servings per large loaf: 18, **per small loaf:** 14
Diabetic exchanges: 1 starch/bread per serving

Sourdough and Variety Breads

ALL ABOUT SOURDOUGH

What is sourdough? It is yeast bread that is leavened by a sourdough starter, or culture, rather than by commercial baker's yeast. The culture contains wild yeast, which produces gas and causes the bread to rise, and bacteria of the genus *Lactobacillus* that give the bread a sour flavor. There are many different sourdough cultures, each with a special flavor of its own and unique rising characteristics.

Perhaps the use of sourdough cultures is beyond the scope of a book dedicated to making bread as easily as possible. However, there are some people who are allergic to commercial baker's yeast and the bread made with it who seem to tolerate sourdough bread. Sourdough bread is not yeast-free; perhaps these people are not allergic to the wild yeast but are allergic to baker's yeast much as one may be allergic to lettuce but not to endive. If you are allergic to yeast, be sure to ask your doctor before trying sourdough bread.

Another reason besides allergies to make your own sourdough bread is for the flavor of the bread itself. If you have eaten at Fisherman's Wharf in San Francisco and are a fan of the sourdough bread there, you may consider the time spent maintaining and using a sourdough culture (or at least using a Lavain du Jour™ starter) worthwhile when you taste how delicious your bread can be.

Some cookbooks contain recipes for making your own sourdough starter. However, in the process of catching and growing wild yeasts from your environment, you may also catch some molds and bacteria that you would rather not have. Also, the flavor of bread made from these homemade starters is barely sour. If you want to make sourdough bread that is really sour, purchase a San Francisco sourdough starter from Sourdoughs International, Inc. (See "Sources," page 212) or some Lavain du Jour™ starter from the King Arthur Flour Baker's Catalogue (See "Sources," page 211). For the best flavor, use your Sourdoughs International starter alone in sourdough bread; never use commercial baker's yeast with it.

Sourdough cultures from Sourdoughs International come with detailed instructions on how to activate and maintain your starter. Activating it involves "feeding" it with flour and water several times and keeping it warm. The dried sourdough culture you receive contains a small amount (less than ¼ cup) of wheat flour. If you wish to make wheat-free bread, feed your culture with white spelt flour or another non-wheat flour. When I activated my cultures, I fed them with white spelt flour nine times before using them in bread. Sparing you the arithmetic, this meant that there was about $\frac{1}{32}$ teaspoon of wheat flour per cup of starter by the time it was first used, or about $\frac{1}{16}$ teaspoon in a large loaf of bread weighing about two pounds. With repeated use and feeding of the culture, the amount of wheat flour continues to decrease, so now I consider my starters to be essentially wheat-free. However, if you are very sensitive to wheat, the flour in the purchased culture may be a problem.

Sourdough bread is a challenge to the bread machine baker because wild yeast takes much longer to leaven bread than commercial baker's yeast and bread machine cycles are based on the way baker's yeast leavens bread. In addition to the wild yeast being slower producers of the gas that makes bread rise, the *lactobacilli* take about twelve hours to develop the full flavor you want in your bread. Also, sourdough cultures are unpredictable, behaving differently from one use to the next. I find it best to use the dough cycle of my bread machine to make the dough and allow the bread to rise outside of the machine where I can easily judge when it is ready to be baked. For further information about sourdough and sourdough bread machine baking, refer to *Worldwide Sourdoughs From Your Bread Machine* by Donna German and Ed Wood.

SOURDOUGH SHORTCUTS

Since the first edition of this book was written, new products have become available which allow you to make "sourdough" bread without keeping and maintaining a traditional sourdough starter. These products are ideal for anyone who wants to make sourdough bread only occasionally.

The easiest-to-use sourdough shortcut is "instant sourdough flavor" which may be purchased from the King Arthur Flour Baker's Catalogue (see "Sources," page 211). This flavor contains corn, rye, and yeast products, but no wheat. Both wheat and wheat-free versions of an instant sourdough bread recipe are included in this chapter. These recipes require just a few hours to make very tasty near-San-Francisco-style sourdough bread with a minimal amount of effort.

If you can eat wheat, you can make sourdough bread which my family says is "like the real San Francisco sourdough" using the LA-4 French sourdough variety of Lavain du Jour™ starter from the King Arthur Flour Baker's Catalogue (see "Sources," page 211). This freeze-dried starter powder is added to each batch of bread and is used along with a small amount of instant yeast. It comes with a recipe and detailed directions for the two to three day process for making bread. If made with King Arthur's artisan bread flour and refrigerated overnight before baking it on the third day, this bread is really sour "like the real thing."

Traditional "San Francisco*" Sourdough Bread

Ingredients:	1½ pound loaf	1 pound loaf
Sourdough culture*	2 cups	1⅓ cups
Bread flour	1½ cups	1 cup
Salt	1 teaspoon	¾ teaspoon
Additional bread flour	2 to 2¾ cups	1⅓ to 1⅞ cups

Cycle: Dough cycle. The night before you want to make bread, mix the culture and the first amount of flour in a glass, plastic, or ceramic mixing bowl. (Do not use a metal bowl). If your bread machine pan does not have a hole in the bottom, mix them in your bread machine pan in the machine. Then cover the bowl or bread machine pan with plastic wrap or a towel and put it in a warm place overnight. (You can easily and inexpensively make a "proofing box" to activate your culture. This is an ideal place to incubate sourdough bread dough. For more information about proofing boxes see page 58 of *The Ultimate Food Allergy Cookbook and Survival Guide* as described on the last pages of this book).

In the morning, put the pan back into the machine or transfer the mixture in the bowl to your machine pan. Add the ingredients below the line in the list above – the salt and the smaller amount of the second flour listed – and start the dough cycle. After mixing, remove the dough from the pan and by hand knead in enough of the remaining flour so the dough is no longer sticky. Shape it into either a round or long loaf and put it on a baking sheet that has been oiled and liberally sprinkled with cornmeal or flour.

Slash the top of the loaf and put it in a warm place to rise until doubled, about 3 to 5 hours. Preheat your oven to 375°F. Spray the loaf with water before baking and at 5 and 10 minutes into the baking time. If desired, bake a few potatoes along with the bread for added moisture to make the crust crisp. Bake for 65 to 80 minutes, or until brown.

*Note: Sourdough International's San Francisco sourdough culture originally came from San Francisco, and bread made with it and this recipe is sour, but if you want "like the real thing" San Francisco sourdough bread, you can make it without maintaining a starter using French Sourdough Lavain du Jour™ starter as described on the previous page.

Nutritional analysis per serving: 79 cal, 2.5 g protein, 16 g carbohydrate, 0.2 g fat, 0 g sat fat, 0 mg
 cholesterol, 72 mg sodium, 0.1 g fiber
Serving size: approximately 1.3 ounce
Servings per large loaf: 22, **per small loaf:**15
Diabetic exchanges: 1 starch/bread per serving

Wheat-Free Traditional "San Francisco" Sourdough Bread

Ingredients:	1½ pound loaf	1 pound loaf
White spelt sourdough culture	2 cups	1⅓ cups
(See pages 94 to 95 about essentially wheat-free cultures).		
White spelt flour	1½ cups	1 cup
Salt	1 teaspoon	¾ teaspoon
Additional white spelt flour	2½ to 3¾ cups	1⅔ to 2½ cups

Cycle: Dough cycle. The night before you want to make bread, mix the culture and the first amount of flour in a glass, plastic, or ceramic mixing bowl. (Do not use a metal bowl). If your bread machine pan does not have a hole in the bottom, mix them in your bread machine pan in the machine. Then cover the bowl or bread machine pan with plastic wrap or a towel and put it in a warm place overnight. (You can easily and inexpensively make a "proofing box" to activate your culture. This is an ideal place to incubate sourdough bread dough. For more information about proofing boxes see page 58 of *The Ultimate Food Allergy Cookbook and Survival Guide* as described on the last pages of this book).

In the morning, put the pan back into the machine or transfer the mixture in the bowl to your machine pan. Add the ingredients below the line in the list above – the salt and the smaller amount of the second flour listed – and start the dough cycle. After mixing, remove the dough from the pan and by hand knead in enough of the remaining flour so the dough is no longer sticky. Shape it into either a round or long loaf and put it on a baking sheet that has been oiled and liberally sprinkled with cornmeal or white spelt flour.

Slash the top of the loaf and put it in a warm place to rise until doubled, about 3 to 5 hours. Preheat your oven to 375°F. Spray the loaf with water before baking and at 5 and 10 minutes into the baking time. If desired, bake a few potatoes along with the bread for added moisture to make the crust crisp. Bake for 65 to 80 minutes, or until brown.

Nutritional analysis per serving: 77 cal, 3.0 g protein, 16 g carbohydrate, 0.4 g fat, 0 g sat fat, 0 mg cholesterol, 72 mg sodium, 0.4 g fiber
Serving size: approximately 1.2 ounce
Servings per large loaf: 28, **per small loaf:** 18
Diabetic exchanges: 1 starch/bread per serving

"Instant Sourdough" Bread

Ingredients: **1½ pound loaf**

    Water   1¼ cups
    Apple juice concentrate, thawed   1½ tablespoons
    Salt   1½ teaspoons
    "Instant sourdough" flavor*   ⅜ cup
    Bread flour   3½ to 3¾ cups
    Active dry yeast**   2¼ teaspoons

Cycle: Dough cycle starting with 3½ cups of flour. This dough softens as it kneads, so check it near the end of the kneading time and add the additional ¼ cup of flour, or more if necessary. At the end of the cycle, shape the dough into a round loaf and put it on a baking sheet that has been oiled and liberally sprinkled with cornmeal or flour.

Slash the top of the loaf and put it in a warm place to rise until doubled, about 30 to 45 minutes. (If you use an extremely sharp knife or lamé to slash the top of your loaf, you may wait until just before baking to slash it). Preheat your oven to 375°F. Spray the loaf with water before baking and at 5 and 10 minutes into the baking time. If desired, bake a few potatoes along with the bread for added moisture to make the crust crisp. Bake for 40 to 55 minutes, or until crusty and very brown.

Notes: *Instant sourdough flavor may be purchased from the King Arthur Flour Baker's Catalogue. See "Sources," page 211.

**SAF Gold™ instant yeast may be substituted for active dry yeast. If you use SAF Gold™, your bread will rise more quickly because this yeast is resistant to the higher acid level of sourdough. SAF Gold™ may be purchased from the King Arthur Flour Baker's Catalogue.

Nutritional analysis per serving: 80 cal, 2.2 g protein, 16.9 g carbohydrate, 0.2 g fat, 0 g sat fat, 0 mg cholesterol, 181 mg sodium, 0.6 g fiber
  Serving size: approximately 1.2 ounce
  Servings per loaf: 22
  Diabetic exchanges: 1 starch/bread per serving

Wheat-Free "Instant Sourdough" Bread

Ingredients: **1½ pound loaf**

Water	1¼ cups
Apple juice concentrate, thawed	1½ tablespoons
Salt	1½ teaspoons
"Instant sourdough" flavor*	⅜ cup
White spelt flour	4½ to 4¾ cups
Active dry yeast**	2¼ teaspoons

Cycle: Dough cycle starting with 4½ cups of flour. This dough softens as it kneads, so check it near the end of the kneading time and add the additional ¼ cup of flour, or more if necessary. At the end of the cycle, shape the dough into a round loaf and put it on a baking sheet that has been oiled and liberally sprinkled with cornmeal or white spelt flour.

Slash the top of the loaf and put it in a warm place to rise until doubled, about 30 to 45 minutes. (If you use an extremely sharp knife or lamé to slash the top of your loaf, you may wait until just before baking to slash it). Preheat your oven to 375°F. Spray the loaf with water before baking and at 5 and 10 minutes into the baking time. If desired, bake a few potatoes along with the bread for added moisture to make the crust crisp. Bake for 40 to 55 minutes, or until crusty and very brown.

Notes: *Instant sourdough flavor may be purchased from the King Arthur Flour Baker's Catalogue. See "Sources," page 211.

** SAF Gold™ instant yeast may be substituted for active dry yeast. If you use SAF Gold™, your bread will rise more quickly because this yeast is resistant to the higher acid level of sourdough. SAF Gold™ may be purchased from the King Arthur Flour Baker's Catalogue.

Nutritional analysis per serving: 78 cal, 3.0 g protein, 16.5 g carbohydrate, 0.4 g fat, 0 g sat fat, 0 mg cholesterol, 181 mg sodium, 0.8 g fiber
Serving size: approximately 1.2 ounce
Servings per loaf: 22
Diabetic exchanges: 1 starch/bread per serving

Easy Sour Rye Bread

Ingredients:	1½ pound loaf	1 pound loaf
Water	1 cup	¾ cup
Apple juice concentrate, thawed	¼ cup	3 tablespoons
Oil	1 tablespoon	2 teaspoons
Liquid lecithin (or may use additional oil)	½ tablespoon	1 teaspoon
Salt	1½ teaspoons	1 teaspoon
Caraway seed (optional)	1 tablespoon	2¼ teaspoons
Heidelberg rye sour*	2 tablespoons	1½ tablespoons
Bread flour	2¼ cups	1⅔ cups
Rye flour	1 cup	¾ cup
Active dry yeast	2¼ teaspoons	1¾ teaspoons

Cycle: Basic yeast bread

*Note: Heidelberg rye sour may be purchased from the King Arthur Flour Baker's Catalogue. See "Sources," page 211.

Nutritional analysis per serving: 81 cal, 1.1 g protein, 15 g carbohydrate, 1.1 g fat, 0 g sat fat, 0 mg cholesterol, 144 mg sodium, 1.0g fiber
Serving size: approximately 1.2 ounce
Servings per large loaf: 21, **per small loaf:** 16
Diabetic exchanges: 1 starch/bread per serving

Onion-Dill Bread

Ingredients:	1½ pound loaf	1 pound loaf
Ingredients for one batch (1 pound or 1½ pound loaf) of any bread, pages 60 to top of 62, 65, 66, 70 to 78, or 81 to 86		
Also add to the bread pan with dry ingredients:		
Dry minced onion	2 teaspoons	1½ teaspoons
Dry dill	2 teaspoons	1½ teaspoons

Cycle: Basic yeast bread cycle, programmable cycle, or dough cycle, the same as in the bread recipe you are using.

Nutritional analysis per serving: Same as for the recipe used
    Serving size and servings per loaf: Same as for the recipe used
    Diabetic exchanges: Same as for the recipe used

Wheat-Free Easy Sour Rye Bread

Ingredients:	1½ pound loaf	1 pound loaf
Water	1 cup	¾ cup
Apple juice concentrate, thawed	¼ cup	3 tablespoons
Oil	1 tablespoon	2 teaspoons
Liquid lecithin (or may use additional oil)	½ tablespoon	1 teaspoon
Salt	1½ teaspoons	1 teaspoon
Caraway seed (optional)	1 tablespoon	2¼ teaspoons
Heidelberg rye sour*	2 tablespoons	1½ tablespoons
White spelt flour	2¾ cups	2 cups + 1 tablespoon
Rye flour	1 cup	¾ cup
Active dry yeast	2¼ teaspoons	1¾ teaspoons

Cycle: Basic yeast bread

*Note: Heidelberg rye sour may be purchased from the King Arthur Flour Baker's Catalogue. See "Sources," page 211.

Nutritional analysis per serving: 81 cal, 2.6 g protein, 15 g carbohydrate, 1.2 g fat, 0 g sat fat, 0 mg cholesterol, 126 mg sodium, 1.0g fiber
    Serving size: approximately 1.1 ounce
    Servings per large loaf: 24, **per small loaf:** 18
    Diabetic exchanges: 1 starch/bread per serving

Chile Corn Bread

Ingredients:	1½ pound loaf	1 pound loaf
Water	⅝ cup	⅜ cup
Apple juice concentrate, thawed	¼ cup	3 tablespoons
4-ounce cans mild green chiles	1 can	1 can
Oil	1 tablespoon	2 teaspoons
Liquid lecithin (or may use additional oil)	½ tablespoon	1 teaspoon
Salt	1 teaspoon	¾ teaspoon
Bread flour	2⅞ cups	2⅛ cups + 1 tablespoon
Cornmeal	⅓ cup	¼ cup
Active dry yeast	1¾ teaspoons	1¼ teaspoons

Cycle: Basic yeast bread

Nutritional analysis per serving: 81cal, 2.1 g protein, 15 g carbohydrate, 1.2 g fat, 0 g sat fat, 0 mg cholesterol, 110 mg sodium, 0.07 g fiber
Serving size: approximately 1.2 ounce
Servings per large loaf: 20, **per small loaf:** 15
Diabetic exchanges: 1 starch/bread per serving

Wheat-Free Chile Corn Bread

Ingredients:	1½ pound loaf	1 pound loaf
Water	⅝ cup	⅜ cup
Apple juice concentrate, thawed	¼ cup	3 tablespoons
4-ounce cans mild green chiles	1 can	1 can
Oil	1 tablespoon	2 teaspoons
Liquid lecithin (or may use additional oil)	½ tablespoon	1 teaspoon
Salt	1 teaspoon	¾ teaspoon
Bread flour	3⅛ cups	2⅓ cups
Cornmeal	⅓ cup	¼ cup
Active dry yeast	1¾ teaspoons	1¼ teaspoons

Cycle: Basic yeast bread

Nutritional analysis per serving: 81 cal, 2.5 g protein, 15 g carbohydrate, 1.2 g fat, 0 g sat fat, 0 mg
cholesterol, 100 mg sodium, 0.3 g fiber
Serving size: approximately 1.2 ounce
Servings per large loaf: 22, **per small loaf:** 17
Diabetic exchanges: 1 starch/bread per serving

Seeded Bread Braid or Ring

Ingredients:	**1½ pound loaf**	**1 pound loaf**

Ingredients for one batch (1 pound or 1½ pound loaf) of any bread on pages 60 to
71, 73 to 81, 84 (kamut only), bottom of 86 to 88, 90, or 92
Bread wash, page 111 OR one slightly beaten egg white
Your choice of two of the following:
 1½ tablespoons sesame seeds
 1½ tablespoons poppy seeds
 2 tablespoons wheat germ

Cycle: Dough cycle. Put the ingredients for the type of bread you have chosen into your
machine and run the dough cycle. When it is finished, for a braid, divide the dough into
three parts and roll each into a 15-inch rope. Lay the ropes on an oiled baking sheet and
braid them. For a ring, divide the dough into two parts and roll each part into a 20-inch to
24-inch rope. Place the ropes side by side near one edge of an oiled baking sheet. Bring the
outer rope across the inner one repeatedly until the ropes are formed into a ring-shaped
twist. Pinch the ends of the ring together. Let the loaf rise until double, about 40 to 60
minutes. Brush it with the wash or egg. Sprinkle one type of seed or the wheat germ on one
section of the twist or braid and another on the next, alternating types. Bake at 375°F for 35
to 45 minutes, covering the loaf with foil for the last 10 minutes if needed to prevent over-
browning.

Nutritional analysis per serving: To the values for the recipe used add about 5 calories, 0.3 grams of
protein, 0.6 grams of carbohydrate, and 0.3 grams of fat.
Serving size and servings per loaf: Same as for the recipe used
Diabetic exchanges: Same as for the recipe used

Blueberry Bread

Ingredients: **1½ pound loaf**   **1 pound loaf**

Ingredients for one batch (1 pound or 1½ pound loaf) of any bread on pages 60 to
   top of 62, 65 to 76, or 81 to 86
Also add to the bread pan when the timer for raisins beeps:
   Dry blueberries   ½ cup   ⅓ cup

Cycle: Basic yeast bread cycle, programmable cycle, or dough cycle, same as in the recipe
you are using. Add the blueberries at the "beep" to add raisins or 5 to 10 minutes before the
last kneading ends.

Nutritional analysis per serving: To the calories per serving, add 8 to10 calories. To the carbohydrate
       per serving add 2 g.
   Serving size and servings per loaf: Same as for the recipe used
   Diabetic exchanges: Same as for the recipe used

Italian Herb Bread

Ingredients: **1½ pound loaf**   **1 pound loaf**

Ingredients for one batch (1 pound or 1½ pound loaf) of any bread on pages 60 to
   top of 62, 65 to 76, or 81 to 86
Also add to the bread pan with dry ingredients:
   Sweet basil, dry   2 teaspoons dry   1½ teaspoons dry
      or minced fresh   OR 2 tablespoons fresh   OR 1½ tbsp. fresh
   Oregano, dry   2 teaspoons dry   1½ teaspoons dry
      or minced fresh   OR 2 tablespoons fresh   OR 1½ tbsp. fresh

Cycle: Basic yeast bread cycle, programmable cycle, or dough cycle, same as in the recipe
you are using.

Nutritional analysis per serving: Same as for the recipe used
   Serving size and servings per loaf: Same as for the recipe used
   Diabetic exchanges: Same as for the recipe used

Poppy Seed Bread

Ingredients: **1½ pound loaf**   **1 pound loaf**

Ingredients for one batch (1 pound or 1½ pound loaf) of any bread, pages 60 to
    top of 62, 65 to 78, or 81 to 86
Also add to the bread pan with dry ingredients:

	1½ pound loaf	1 pound loaf
Poppy seeds	2 tablespoons	1½ tablespoons

Cycle: Basic yeast bread cycle, programmable cycle, or dough cycle, same as in the recipe you are using.

Nutritional analysis per serving: Add 4 cal and 0.5 g fat to each serving. Saturated fat stays the same.
    Serving size and servings per loaf: Same as for the recipe used
    Diabetic exchanges: Same as for the recipe used

Herb Focaccia

Ingredients:

One batch of "Italian Bread" OR "Wheat-free Italian Bread" dough, pages 62 to 63
4 teaspoons olive oil
2 to 3 tablespoons minced fresh sweet basil or rosemary
    OR 2 to 3 teaspoons dry sweet basil or rosemary

Cycle: Dough cycle, using only the Italian bread ingredients, not the oil and herbs. When the cycle is finished, remove the dough from the machine and divide it in half. Spray two baking sheets with a cooking oil spray or oil them lightly. Roll out each piece of dough on a baking sheet to an 8-inch to 10-inch circle about ½ inch thick. Brush each circle with 2 teaspoons of olive oil and sprinkle with the herbs. Let rise in a warm place for 30 minutes or until double in volume. Bake at 375°F for 20 to 25 minutes or until brown. Cut into wedges to serve.

Nutritional analysis per serving: Add 8 to 10 calories and 1 gram of fat to the values for the recipe used
    Serving size and servings per batch: Same as for the recipe used
    Diabetic exchanges: Same as for the recipe used

Salt and Pepper Focaccia

Make as for "Herb Focaccia" on the previous page except substitute ½ teaspoon kosher salt and ¼ teaspoon pepper for the herbs.

Nutritional analysis per serving: Add 8 to 10 calories, 1 g fat, and 50 mg sodium to the values for the bread recipe used
    Serving size and servings per batch: Same as for the recipe used
    Diabetic exchanges: Same as for the recipe used

Pita Bread

Ingredients:

One 1½-pound-loaf batch of dough made with "White Bread" recipe, page 60

Cycle: Dough cycle. After the cycle is finished, remove the dough from the machine and preheat your oven to 475°F. Roll the dough out on a very lightly oiled board with an oiled rolling pin to about ¼ inch thickness. Fold the dough in half and roll it to ¼ inch thickness again. Fold and roll it repeatedly until you have rolled it 15 to 20 times, letting the dough "rest" for five minutes after each set of five rollings. Divide the dough into eight pieces and allow the dough to rest for five minutes. Roll each piece out into a 6 inch to 7 inch circle, flouring both sides of the circle as you roll it. Place the pita breads on lightly floured baking sheets and bake them in the preheated oven until they are lightly browned, about 3 to 9 minutes. Remove them from the oven and immediately wrap them in a very lightly dampened dishcloth. When they are completely cool, remove them from the dishcloth and store them in a plastic bag. Use a serrated knife to cut them in half and open any places where the top and bottom of the pita did not separate.

Nutritional analysis per serving: 195 cal, 5.4 g protein, 36 g carbohydrate, 2.8 g fat, 0 g sat fat, 0 mg cholesterol, 254 mg sodium, 0.1 g fiber
    Serving size: one pita bread (or eat ½ pita bread for half of the calories, carbs, and exchanges)
    Servings per batch: 8 pita breads
    Diabetic exchanges: 2½ starch/bread per serving

White Spelt Pita Bread

Ingredients:

One 1½-pound-loaf batch of dough made with "White Spelt Bread" recipe, page 61

Cycle: Dough cycle. After the cycle is finished, remove the dough from the machine and preheat your oven to 475°F. Roll the dough out on a very lightly oiled board with an oiled rolling pin to about ¼ inch thickness. Fold the dough in half and roll it to ¼ inch thickness again. Fold and roll it repeatedly until you have rolled it 15 to 20 times. Divide the dough into eight pieces. Roll each piece out into a 6-inch to 7-inch circle, flouring both sides of the circle as you roll it. Place the pita breads on lightly floured baking sheets and bake them in the preheated oven until they are lightly browned, about 3 to 7 minutes. Remove them from the oven and immediately wrap them in a very lightly dampened dishcloth. When they are completely cool, remove them from the dishcloth and store them in a plastic bag. Use a serrated knife to cut them in half and open any places where the top and bottom of the pita did not separate.

Nutritional analysis per serving: 179 cal, 6.0 g protein, 33 g carbohydrate, 2.6 g fat, 0 g sat fat, 0 mg cholesterol, 191 mg sodium, 0.7 g fiber
Serving size: one pita bread (or eat ½ pita bread for half of the calories, carbs, and exchanges)
Servings per batch: 8 pita breads
Diabetic exchanges: 2¼ starch/bread per serving

Whole Wheat Pita Bread

Ingredients:

One 1½-pound-loaf batch of dough made with "100% Whole Wheat Bread" recipe, page 74

Cycle: Dough cycle. After the cycle is finished, remove the dough from the machine and preheat your oven to 475°F. Roll the dough out on a very lightly oiled board with an oiled rolling pin to about ¼ inch thickness. Fold the dough in half and roll it to ¼ inch thickness again. Fold and roll it repeatedly until you have rolled it 15 to 20 times. Divide the dough into ten pieces. Roll each piece out into a 5-inch to 6-inch circle, flouring both sides of the circle as you roll it. Place the pita breads on lightly floured baking sheets and bake them in the preheated oven until they are lightly browned, about 7 to 11 minutes. Remove them from the oven and immediately wrap them in a very lightly dampened dishcloth. When they are completely cool, remove them from the dishcloth and store them in a plastic bag. Use a serrated knife to cut them in half and open any places where the top and bottom of the pita did not separate.

Nutritional analysis per serving: 211 cal, 7.0 g protein, 38 g carbohydrate, 3.3 g fat, 0 g sat fat, 0 mg cholesterol, 205 mg sodium, 1.2 g fiber
Serving size: one pita bread (or eat ½ pita bread for half of the calories, carbs, and exchanges)
Servings per batch: 10 pita breads
Diabetic exchanges: 2½ starch/bread per serving

Whole Spelt Pita Bread

Ingredients:

One 1½-pound-loaf batch of dough made with "Whole Grain Spelt Bread" recipe, page 76

Cycle: Dough cycle. After the cycle is finished, remove the dough from the machine and preheat your oven to 475°F. Roll the dough out on a very lightly oiled board with an oiled rolling pin to about ¼ inch thickness. Fold the dough in half and roll it to ¼ inch thickness again. Fold and roll it repeatedly until you have rolled it 15 to 20 times. Divide the dough into eight pieces. Roll each piece out into a 6-inch to 7-inch circle, flouring both sides of the circle as you roll it. Place the pita breads on lightly floured baking sheets and bake them in the preheated oven until they are lightly browned, about 5 to 9 minutes. Remove them from the oven and immediately wrap them in a very lightly dampened dishcloth. When they are completely cool, remove them from the dishcloth and store them in a plastic bag. Use a serrated knife to cut them in half and open any places where the top and bottom of the pita did not separate.

Nutritional analysis per serving: 218 cal, 7.0 g protein, 39 g carbohydrate, 3.8 g fat, 0 g sat fat, 0 mg cholesterol, 192 mg sodium, 3.4 g fiber
Serving size: one pita bread (or eat ½ pita bread for half of the calories, carbs, and exchanges)
Servings per batch: 8 pita breads
Diabetic exchanges: 2¾ starch/bread per serving

Rolls and Buns

Descriptions of special holidays and meals often include memories of freshly baked rolls or buns. Now you can make fresh buns or rolls easily for any special occasion. Fresh homemade rolls take little effort to make using your bread machine with the recipes in this chapter and the sweet rolls chapter, page 197.

Individual preference may determine the size of the rolls or buns that you make. Also, many of the recipes in this chapter begin with a choice of dough made from bread recipes in other chapters. This makes it challenging to produce standard nutritional information for each roll and bun recipe! If you need this information, you will have to do a little math. Multiply the nutritional values per serving times the number of servings in a loaf of bread for the batch size of the dough you are making. This will give you the calories, grams of protein, etc. for the whole batch of dough. (Whole-batch values are included with the roll dough recipes on the next few pages and in the sweet rolls chapter). Add the nutritional values for the whole batch of dough to the values for any other ingredients included in the roll recipes. (This information is found at the end of each roll recipe). Then divide the totals by the number of rolls you made.

Enjoy these rolls and buns, and make some special memories!

Basic Roll or Bun Dough

Ingredients: **1, 1½, or 2 pound machine**

Water	⅞ cup
Apple juice concentrate, thawed	¼ cup
Oil	1 tablespoon
Liquid lecithin (or use additional oil)	½ tablespoon
Salt	1 teaspoon
Bread flour	3⅛ cups
Active dry yeast	1¾ teaspoons

Cycle: Dough cycle. Shape and bake as in the recipes on pages 112 to the top of 120.

Nutritional analysis per batch: 1557 cal, 43 g protein, 286 g carbohydrate, 23 g fat, 0 g sat fat, 0 mg
        cholesterol, 2031 mg sodium, 0.9 g fiber
Nutritional analysis per roll if you make 15 rolls: 104 cal, 2.9 g protein, 19 g carbohydrate, 1.5 g fat, 0 g
        sat fat, 0 mg cholesterol, 135 mg sodium, 0.06 g fiber
    Serving size: approximately 1.5 ounces if you make 15 rolls
    Servings per batch: 15 for the per roll nutritional values above
    Diabetic exchanges: 1¼ starch/bread per roll if you make 15 rolls
                          1½ starch/bread per roll if you make 12 rolls
                          1 starch/bread per roll if you make 19 small rolls

Gluten-Free Basic Roll or Bun Dough

Ingredients: 1, 1½, or 2 pound machine

Water	½ cup + 1 tablespoon
Apple juice concentrate, thawed	¼ cup
Oil	2 tablespoons
Eggs OR egg substitute	3 eggs OR ¾ cup egg substitute
Salt	1 teaspoon
Vitamin C crystals	⅛ teaspoon
Guar gum	4 teaspoons
Brown rice flour	2 cups
Potato flour	⅓ cup
Tapioca flour	⅓ cup
Active dry yeast	2¼ teaspoons

Cycle: Dough cycle. Shape and bake as in the recipes where included in the ingredient list
on pages 112 to 120.

Nutritional analysis per batch made with eggs: 1891 cal, 54 g protein, 325 g carbohydrate, 52 g fat, 5.1
        g sat fat, 1029 mg cholesterol, 2286 mg sodium, 17 g fiber
Nutritional analysis per roll made with eggs if you make 16 rolls: 118 cal, 3.4 g protein, 20 g carbohy-
        drate, 3.2 g fat, 0.4 g sat fat, 64 mg cholesterol, 143 mg sodium, 1.1 g fiber
Nutritional analysis per batch made with egg substitute: 1883 cal, 54 g protein, 325 g carbohydrate,
        61 g fat, 0 g sat fat, 0 mg cholesterol, 2361 mg sodium, 17 g fiber
Nutritional analysis per roll made with egg substitute if you make 16 rolls: 118 cal, 3.4 g protein, 20 g
        carbohydrate, 3.8 g fat, 0 g sat fat, 0 mg cholesterol, 148 mg sodium, 1.1 g fiber
    Serving size: approximately 1.6 ounces if you make 16 rolls
    Servings per batch: 16 for the per roll nutritional values above
    Diabetic exchanges: 1½ starch/bread per roll if you make 16 rolls
                          1 starch/bread per roll if you make 24 small rolls

Wheat-Free Basic Roll or Bun Dough

Ingredients:	1, 1½, or 2 pound machine
Water	⅞ cup
Apple juice concentrate, thawed	¼ cup
Oil	1 tablespoon
Liquid lecithin (or may use additional oil)	½ tablespoon
Salt	1 teaspoon
White spelt flour	3½ cups
Active dry yeast	1¾ teaspoons

Cycle: Dough cycle. Shape and bake as in the recipes on pages 112 to the top of 120.

Nutritional analysis per batch: 1708 cal, 56 g protein, 314 g carbohydrate, 24 g fat, 0 g sat fat, 0 mg cholesterol, 2031 mg sodium, 7 g fiber
Nutritional analysis per roll if you make 16 rolls: 107 cal, 3.5 g protein, 20 g carbohydrate, 1.5 g fat, 0 g sat fat, 0 mg cholesterol, 127 mg sodium, 0.4 g fiber
   Serving size: approximately 1.4 ounces if you make 16 rolls
   Servings per batch: 16 for the per roll nutritional values above
   Diabetic exchanges: 1¼ starch/bread per roll if you make 16 rolls
                   1¾ starch/bread per roll if you make 12 rolls
                   1 starch/bread per roll if you make 21 small rolls

Bread or Bun Wash

Brush this on your bread or buns instead of egg white to make the crust shiny and help seeds or other toppings stick.

¼ cup water
1 teaspoon tapioca flour or cornstarch

Combine the water and starch in a small saucepan, bring them to a boil, reduce the heat, and simmer until the mixture is clear and the consistency of egg white. Or, combine the water and starch in a glass container and microwave them for 45 seconds to 1 minute, stirring every 15 seconds. Allow the wash to cool to lukewarm. Brush it on bread or buns after shaping them and sprinkle with seeds if desired. Allow them to rise and bake as directed in the bread or bun recipe.

Nutritional analysis for the whole batch: 10 calories, 2.5 g carbohydrate

Hot Dog Buns

Ingredients:

1 batch of dough made with any of the following recipes:
    Any Basic Roll or Bun Dough, pages 109 to 111
    Any 1½ pound batch of dough made with a basic bread recipe, pages 60 to 71
    Any 1½ pound batch of dough made with a whole grain bread recipe, pages 73 to
        78, 81, top of 84, bottom of 86 to 88, 90, or 92
Cooking oil spray or cooking oil

Cycle: Dough cycle. When the cycle has finished, divide the dough into 12 pieces. Spray with cooking oil spray or lightly oil three 8-inch or 9-inch square pans or two 13-inch by 9-inch pans. (For the rice dough, oil two square pans and divide the dough into 8 pieces). Roll the pieces of dough into ropes that are about 7-inch to 8-inch long, and line them up parallel to each other in the pans. (Put 4 in each square pan or 6 in each rectangular pan). Allow them to rise for 30 to 45 minutes, or until they have doubled in volume. Bake at 375°F for 15 to 20 minutes, or until browned. Remove them from the pans and put them on racks immediately. Break them apart into individual buns when they are cool.

Nutritional analysis per serving: Divide the whole batch values for the bread or dough recipe used by 12 or the number of buns you made.
Diabetic exchanges: Divide the total number of exchanges per batch of the recipe you used by the number of buns you made.

Hamburger Buns

Ingredients:

1 batch of dough made with any of the following recipes:
    Basic Roll or Bun Dough, page 109
    Wheat-free Basic Roll or Bun Dough, page 111
    Any 1½ pound batch of dough made with a basic bread recipe, pages 60 to 71
    Any 1½ pound batch of dough made with a whole grain bread recipe, pages 73 to
        78, 81, top of 84, bottom of 86 to 88, top of 90, or 92
Cooking oil spray or cooking oil

Cycle: Dough cycle. When the cycle has finished, divide the dough into 12 pieces, or the number necessary to make buns of the size you desire. Spray a baking sheet with cooking oil spray or lightly oil it. Knead the pieces of dough briefly, form them into balls, and put them on the baking sheet. Allow them to rise for 30 to 45 minutes, or until they have doubled in volume. Bake at 375°F for 13 to 18 minutes, or until browned.

Nutritional analysis per serving: Divide the whole batch values for the bread or dough recipe used by 12 or the number of buns you made.
Diabetic exchanges: Divide the total number of exchanges per batch of the recipe you used by the number of buns you made.

Onion Rolls or Buns

These buns are great with hamburgers.

Ingredients:

1 batch of dough made with any of the following recipes:
 Basic Roll or Bun Dough, page 109
 Wheat-free Basic Roll or Bun Dough, page 111
 Any 1½ pound batch of dough made with a basic bread recipe, pages 60 to 71
 Any 1½ pound batch of dough made with a whole grain bread recipe, pages 73 to 78, 81, top of 84, bottom of 86 to 88, top of 90, or 92
2 tablespoons dried minced onion, divided
2 tablespoons water
1 slightly beaten egg white or "Bread or Bun Wash," page 111

Cycle: Dough cycle. Add 1 tablespoon of the onion to the dough with the salt when you start the machine. While the cycle is running, soak the remaining 1 tablespoon of onion in the water for 15 minutes; then drain it on paper towel. When the cycle is finished, shape 16 rolls or 12 hamburger buns as on page 112. Brush them with the egg white or wash and sprinkle them with the drained onion. Allow them to rise for 30 to 45 minutes, or until they have doubled in volume. Bake at 375°F for 13 to 18 minutes, or until browned.

Nutritional analysis per serving: To the whole batch values for the bread or dough recipe used add 28 calories and 7 g carbohydrate. Divide the totals by the number of buns you made.
Diabetic exchanges: Divide the total number of exchanges per batch of the recipe you used by the number of buns you made.

Poppy or Sesame Seed Rolls or Buns

Ingredients:

1 batch of dough made with any of the following recipes:
  Any Basic Roll or Bun Dough, pages 109 to 111
  Any 1½ pound batch of dough made with a basic bread recipe, pages 60 to 71
  Any 1½ pound batch of dough made with a whole grain bread recipe, pages 73 to 78, 81, top of 84, bottom of 86 to 88, 90, or 92
1 slightly beaten egg white or "Bread or Bun Wash," page 111
1 tablespoon poppy seeds or sesame seeds

Cycle: Dough cycle. When the cycle has finished, shape the rolls as directed in the your choice of the roll recipes on pages 112, 116, or 118 through 120. Brush them with the egg white or wash, and sprinkle with the poppy or sesame seeds. Allow them to rise and bake them as directed in the roll or bun recipe.

Nutritional analysis per serving if made with poppy seeds: To the whole batch values for the bread or dough recipe used add 15 calories and 1.5 g fat. Divide the totals by 12 or the number of buns you made.
Nutritional analysis per serving if made with sesame seeds: To the whole batch values for the bread or dough recipe used add 25 calories, 2 g protein, and 1.5 g fat. Divide the totals by 12 or the number of buns you made.
Diabetic exchanges: Divide the total number of exchanges per batch of the recipe you used by the number of buns you made.

Cornmeal Rolls

Ingredients:

1 batch of dough made with any of the following recipes:
  White Corn Bread, page 68
  Wheat-free White Corn Bread, page 69
  Corny Bread, page 92
  Wheat-free Corny Bread, page 92
  Gluten-free Corny Bread, page 93

Cycle: Dough cycle. When the cycle is finished, knead the dough (except for the gluten-free dough) briefly and form it into 9 to 12 balls. Spray a muffin tin with cooking oil spray or lightly oil it. Place each ball in a muffin cup. For the gluten-free dough, spoon enough dough into each muffin cup to fill it ⅔ full. Allow the rolls to rise until double in volume, 40 to 60 minutes. Bake at 375°F for 15 to 20 minutes, or until brown.

Nutritional analysis per serving: Divide the whole batch values for the recipe you used by the number of rolls you made.
Diabetic exchanges: Divide the total number of exchanges per batch of the recipe you used by the number of rolls you made.

Cinnamon Roll-Ups

Ingredients:

    1 batch of dough made with any of the following recipes:
        Basic Roll or Bun Dough, page 109
        Wheat-free Basic Roll or Bun Dough, page 111
        Any 1½ pound batch of dough made with a basic bread recipe, pages 60 to 71
        Any 1½ pound batch of dough made with a whole grain bread recipe, pages 73 to 78, 81, top of 84, bottom of 86 to 88, top of 90, or 92
    Cooking oil spray or cooking oil
    ¼ cup date sugar (optional)
    Cinnamon (optional)

Cycle: Dough cycle. After the cycle is finished, knead the dough briefly on a lightly oiled board. Spray a baking sheet with cooking oil spray or lightly oil it. Roll the dough out with an oiled rolling pin into a circle ⅛-inch thick to ¼-inch thick. If desired, sprinkle the dough with the optional cinnamon or cinnamon and date sugar. Cut the circle into quarters and each quarter into 3 to 4 pieces like pie wedges so you end up with 12 to 16 triangular pieces of dough. Spray the pieces with cooking oil spray or brush them lightly with oil. Roll each wedge up, starting at the wide end. Put them on the baking sheet with the point of the wedge on the bottom of the roll. Allow to rise until double in volume, about 30 to 40 minutes. Bake at 375°F for 15 to 25 minutes, or until lightly browned.

Nutritional analysis per serving: If the date sugar is used, add 64 cal,16 g carbohydrates and 2 g fiber to the whole batch values for the dough recipe used. Divide totals by the number of rolls you made.
Diabetic exchanges: Divide the total number of exchanges per batch of the recipe you used by the number of rolls you made.

Fan-Tans

Ingredients:

1 batch of dough made with any of the following recipes:
    Basic Roll or Bun Dough, page 109
    Wheat-free Basic Roll or Bun Dough, page 111
    Any 1½ pound batch of dough made with a basic bread recipe, pages 60 to 71
    Any 1½ pound batch of dough made with a whole grain bread recipe, pages 73 to
        78, 81, top of 84, bottom of 86 to 88, top of 90, or 92
Cooking oil spray or cooking oil

Cycle: Dough cycle. After the cycle is finished, knead the dough briefly on a lightly oiled board. Spray a muffin tin with cooking oil spray or lightly oil it. Roll the dough out with an oiled rolling pin to ⅛-inch to ¼-inch thickness. Cut it into strips 1½ inches wide. Stack 6 to 7 strips, spraying with cooking oil spray or brushing lightly with oil between layers. Cut the stacks of strips into 1½-inch segments, and put a stack of several squares of dough into each muffin cup with the cut edges of the squares up. Allow to rise until double in volume, about 30 to 40 minutes, and bake at 375°F for 15 to 25 minutes, or until lightly browned.

Nutritional analysis per serving: Divide the whole batch values for the recipe you used by the number of rolls you made.
Diabetic exchanges: Divide the total number of exchanges per batch of the recipe you used by the number of rolls you made.

Cloverleaf Rolls

Ingredients:

1 batch of dough made with any of the following recipes:
    Any Basic Roll or Bun Dough, pages 109 to 111
    Any 1½ pound batch of dough made with a basic bread recipe, pages 60 to 71
    Any 1½ pound batch of dough made with a whole grain bread recipe, pages 73 to
        78, 81, top of 84, bottom of 86 to 88, top of 90, or 92
Cooking oil spray or cooking oil

Cycle: Dough cycle. After the cycle is finished, knead the dough briefly on a lightly oiled board. Spray a muffin tin with cooking oil spray or lightly oil it. Shape the dough into 1-inch balls. Put three balls into each muffin cup. Allow to rise until double in volume, about 30 to 40 minutes. Bake at 375°F for 15 to 25 minutes, or until lightly browned.

Nutritional analysis per serving: Divide the whole batch values for the recipe you used by the number of rolls you made.

Diabetic exchanges: Divide the total number of exchanges per batch of the recipe you used by the number of rolls you made.

Heart-Healthy Crescent Rolls

Ingredients:

1 batch of dough made with any of the following recipes:
>   Basic Roll or Bun Dough, page 109
>   Wheat-free Basic Roll or Bun Dough, page 111
>   Any 1½ pound batch of dough made with a basic bread recipe, pages 60 to 71
>   Any 1½ pound batch of dough made with a whole grain bread recipe, pages 73 to
>   78, 81, top of 84, bottom of 86 to 88, top of 90, or 92
> Cooking oil spray or cooking oil

Cycle: Dough cycle. After the cycle is finished, knead the dough briefly on a lightly oiled board. Spray a baking sheet with cooking oil spray or lightly oil it. Roll the dough out with an oiled rolling pin into a 12-inch to 15-inch square about ¼-inch thick. Lightly spray the dough with cooking oil spray or brush with cooking oil. Fold it in thirds by folding the right third of the dough over the center third, and then folding the left third over both. Roll the dough to ¼-inch thickness again. Turn the dough 90°, spray or brush it with cooking oil, fold it in thirds and roll it to ¼-inch thickness again. Repeat the spraying or brushing, folding, rolling, and turning process twice more. Roll the dough out into a 12-inch square. Cut off the edges and cut the large square into nine 4-inch squares. Cut each small square diagonally into a triangle. Starting with one of the short sides, roll up each triangle and put it on the baking sheet with the point under the roll, curving it slightly to form a crescent. Allow it to rise in a warm place for 30 to 40 minutes. Bake at 375°F for 15 to 20 minutes.

Nutritional analysis per serving: Divide the whole batch values for the recipe you used by 18 or the number of rolls you made.

Diabetic exchanges: Divide the total number of exchanges per batch of the recipe you used by 18 or the number of rolls you made.

Parker House Rolls

Ingredients:

1 batch of dough made with any of the following recipes:
    Basic Roll or Bun Dough, page 109
    Wheat-free Basic Roll or Bun Dough, page 111
    Any 1½ pound batch of dough made with a basic bread recipe, pages 60 to 71
    Any 1½ pound batch of dough made with a whole grain bread recipe, pages 73 to
        78, 81, top of 84, bottom of 86 to 88, top of 90, or 92
Cooking oil spray or cooking oil

Cycle: Dough cycle. After the cycle is finished, remove the dough from the machine; do not knead it. Spray a baking sheet with cooking oil spray or lightly oil it. Roll the dough out with a lightly oiled rolling pin to ½-inch thickness. Cut it into 2½-inch to 3-inch rounds with a biscuit cutter. Make a deep crease down the center of each round with the handle of a knife. Fold the round over at the crease and press the edges together lightly. Put the rolls on the baking sheet and allow them to rise until double in volume, about 30 to 40 minutes. Bake at 375°F for 15 to 25 minutes, or until lightly browned.

Nutritional analysis per serving: Divide the whole batch values for the recipe you used by the number of rolls you made.
Diabetic exchanges: Divide the total number of exchanges per batch of the recipe you used by the number of rolls you made.

Pan Rolls

Ingredients:

1 batch of dough made with any of the following recipes:
    Any Basic Roll or Bun Dough, pages 109 to 111
    Any 1½ pound batch of dough made with a basic bread recipe, pages 60 to 71
    Any 1½ pound batch of dough made with a whole grain bread recipe, pages 73 to
        78, 81, top of 84, bottom of 86 to 88, 90, or 92
Cooking oil spray or cooking oil

Cycle: Dough cycle. After the cycle is finished, remove the dough from the machine. Knead it briefly on an oiled board. Spray a 9-inch by 13-inch baking pan with cooking oil spray or lightly oil it. Divide the dough into 15 balls. Spray the balls with cooking oil spray or brush them lightly with oil. Put them into the prepared pan in a grid of three rows and five columns. Allow them to rise until double in volume, about 25 to 40 minutes. Bake at 375°F for 25 to 35 minutes, or until lightly browned. Spray them with cooking oil spray or brush them lightly with oil immediately after removing them from the oven.

Nutritional analysis per serving: Divide the whole batch values for the recipe you used by 15 or the number of rolls you made.
Diabetic exchanges: Divide the total number of exchanges per batch of the recipe you used by 15 or the number of rolls you made.

Boolots

My mother once made rolls for a family celebration that came out so large that my grandfather called them "big balls" in Italian. The word, which sounded like "boolots," is what we call large rolls such as these to this day.

Ingredients:

1 batch of dough made with any of the following recipes:
    Any Basic Roll or Bun Dough, pages 109 to 111
    Any 1½ pound batch of dough made with a basic bread recipe, pages 60 to 71
    Any 1½ pound batch of dough made with a whole grain bread recipe, pages 73 to
        78, 81, top of 84, bottom of 86 to 88, 90, or 92
Cooking oil spray or cooking oil

Cycle: Dough cycle. When the cycle is finished, knead the dough briefly and form it into 6 to 8 balls. Spray a "Texas size" muffin tin with cooking oil spray or lightly oil it. Place each ball in a muffin cup. Allow the rolls to rise until double in volume, 40 to 50 minutes. Bake at 375°F until brown, about 20 to 25 minutes.

Nutritional analysis per serving: Divide the whole batch values for the recipe you used by the number of rolls you made.
Diabetic exchanges: Divide the total number of exchanges per batch of the recipe you used by the number of rolls you made.

Dinner Rolls

Ingredients:

1 batch of dough made with any of the following recipes:
    Any Basic Roll or Bun Dough, pages 109 to 111
    Any 1½ pound batch of dough made with a basic bread recipe, pages 60 to 71
    Any 1½ pound batch of dough made with a whole grain bread recipe, pages 73 to
        78, 81, top of 84, bottom of 86 to 88, 90, or 92
Cooking oil spray or cooking oil

Cycle: Dough cycle. When the cycle is finished, knead the dough briefly and form it into 12 to 16 balls. Spray a muffin tin with cooking oil spray or lightly oil it. Place each ball in a muffin cup. Allow the rolls to rise until double in volume, 30 to 50 minutes. Bake at 375°F until brown, 15 to 20 minutes.

Nutritional analysis per serving: Divide the whole batch values for the recipe you used by the number of rolls you made.
Diabetic exchanges: Divide the total number of exchanges per batch of the recipe you used by the number of rolls you made.

Gluten-Free or Low Gluten Rolls or Buns

Low gluten dough needs a pan to maintain its shape as buns. If you make these buns in custard cups or a "Texas size" muffin pan and slice them in half horizontally, they make great hamburger buns.

Ingredients:

1 batch of dough made with any of the following recipes:
    Gluten-free Roll or Bun Dough, page 110
    Amaranth Bread, page 82
    Buckwheat Bread, page 82
    Quinoa Bread, page 83
    No-egg Brown Rice Bread, page 84
    Barley Bread, page 85

Oat Bread, page 86
Gluten-free Corny Bread, page 93

Cycle: Dough cycle. Spray with cooking oil spray or lightly oil a muffin tin, Texas size muffin tin, or custard cups. When the cycle is finished, put the dough into muffin cups, filling them ⅔ full for rolls. Or to make hamburger buns, fill them ⅓ to ½ full. Allow them to rise until barely doubled, 20 to 40 minutes. Bake at 375°F for 15 to 25 minutes, or until browned.

Nutritional analysis per serving: Divide the whole batch values for the recipe you used by the number of rolls you made.
Diabetic exchanges: Divide the total number of exchanges per batch of the recipe you used by the number of rolls you made.

Savory Snails

Ingredients:	**1, 1½, or 2 pound machine**
Water	⅞ cup
Apple juice concentrate, thawed	¼ cup
Oil	1 tablespoon
Liquid lecithin (or may use additional oil)	½ tablespoon
Salt	¾ teaspoon
Bread flour	3⅛ cups
Active dry yeast	1¾ teaspoons
Dried tomato flakes or dried tomatoes cut into ¼-inch pieces	⅓ cup
Additional oil	2 teaspoons
Grated Romano cheese	¼ to ⅓ cup

Cycle: Dough cycle. Add the ingredients above the dotted line to your machine and start the cycle. About 10 minutes before the last kneading time will finish, add the tomatoes. After the cycle finishes, roll the dough out on a lightly oiled board to a 12-inch by 16-inch rectangle. Brush with the additional oil and sprinkle with the cheese. Starting with the long side, roll the dough up like a jelly roll and pinch the edge to the roll. Cut it into 15 slices. Put them cut side down into oiled muffin pans and allow to rise until double, about 30 minutes. Bake at 375°F for 15 to 20 minutes, or until nicely browned.

Nutritional analysis per serving: 120 cal, 3.8 g protein, 20 g carbohydrate, 2.7 g fat, 0.2 g sat fat, 1.3 mg cholesterol, 137 mg sodium, 0.3 g fiber
    Serving size: approximately 1.5 ounce
    Servings per batch: 15
    Diabetic exchanges: 1½ starch/bread per serving

Wheat-Free Savory Snails

Ingredients:	**1, 1½, or 2 pound machine**
Water	⅞ cup
Apple juice concentrate, thawed	¼ cup
Oil	1 tablespoon
Liquid lecithin (or may use additional oil)	½ tablespoon
Salt	¾ teaspoon
White spelt flour	3⅜ cups
Active dry yeast	1¾ teaspoons
Dried tomato flakes or dried tomatoes cut into ¼-inch pieces	⅓ cup
Additional oil	2 teaspoons
Grated Romano cheese	¼ to ⅓ cup

Cycle: Dough cycle. Add the ingredients above the dotted line to your machine and start the cycle. About 10 minutes before the last kneading time will finish, add the tomatoes. After the cycle finishes, roll the dough out on a lightly oiled board to a 12-inch by 16-inch rectangle. Brush with the additional oil and sprinkle with the cheese. Starting with the long side, roll the dough up like a jelly roll and pinch the edge to the roll. Cut it into 15 slices. Put them cut side down into oiled muffin pans and allow to rise until double, about 30 minutes. Bake at 375°F for 15 to 20 minutes, or until nicely browned.

Nutritional analysis per serving: 130 cal, 4.7 g protein, 22 g carbohydrate, 2.8 g fat, 0.2 g sat fat, 1.3 mg cholesterol, 137 mg sodium, 0.7 g fiber
    Serving size: approximately 1.5 ounce
    Servings per batch: 15
    Diabetic exchanges: 1½ starch/bread per serving

No-Yeast Quick Breads and Cakes

Although quick breads are easy to make by hand, if you are on a yeast-free or low yeast diet and eat quick breads exclusively, it is certainly nice to have a machine do most of the work of making it for you. Using your machine's quick bread or cake cycle and the recipes in this chapter, you can have delicious bread for your special diet made with little effort.

Making quick breads or cakes with a bread machine differs from making them by hand and from making yeast breads in a machine in several ways. The first is that you do not add all the liquid ingredients to the dry ingredients at the same time, as you do in making them by hand. Add the oil first, at three to four minutes before your machine will begin baking the bread. Then, about two minutes before the machine will stop mixing and proceed to the baking part of the cycle, add the water and other liquids. During the final two minutes of mixing, you will have to "assist" the mixing more than you normally would assist your machine in mixing yeast breads.

STANDARD MIXING INSTRUCTIONS FOR BREAD MACHINE QUICK BREADS AND CAKES: Put the flour(s), baking powder, and salt (and baking soda, guar gum, spices, and other dry ingredients, if used) in the bread machine. Press "start" and mix for one-half to one minute. (Begin timing AFTER the fast mixing starts if your machine mixes slowly at first). Add the oil and mix for 1 minute. Add the remaining liquid ingredient(s). If the dough is not evenly distributed in the pan at the end of the mixing time, reach in with a rubber spatula and gently spread it so it covers the bottom of the pan fairly evenly. Scrape down the sides of the pan if necessary.

If your machine mixes quickly longer than three to four minutes, the gas produced by the leavening in your bread may all be dissipated before it can be baked into the dough. Therefore, you need to delay starting the action of the leavening ingredients by delaying adding the water or other non-oil liquids that will dissolve the baking soda and acid component in the baking powder until two minutes before the mixing ends and baking begins.

If your machine mixes longer than four minutes, you may add the oil several minutes before it will start baking. The crucial factor in having it rise properly is to delay adding the other liquid ingredients until about two minutes before the end of the mixing time. For example, if it mixes for six minutes, rather than adding the non-oil liquids about two minutes into the cycle, wait until four minutes after you start the machine.

To make quick breads with a large capacity machine which has a rectangular rather than a square-bottomed pan (including the Zojirushi BBCC-V20 and BBCC-X20), multiply the amounts of all the ingredients in the recipes in this chapter by 1½ to 2 to produce a loaf of normal height.

No-Yeast White Bread

Ingredients:

3 cups all-purpose flour
3 teaspoons baking powder
½ teaspoon salt
¼ cup oil
1¼ cups water

Cycle: Quick bread or cake cycle. Add ingredients to the pan as described and assist the mixing as directed in the standard mixing instructions for quick breads on page 123.

Nutritional analysis per serving: 80 cal, 1.7 g protein, 12 g carbohydrate, 2.7 g fat, 0 g sat fat, 0 mg cholesterol, 111 mg sodium, 0.04 g fiber
   Serving size: approximately 1.1 ounce
   Servings per loaf: 21
   Diabetic exchanges: 1 starch/bread per serving

No-Yeast White Spelt Bread

Ingredients:

3 cups white spelt flour
3 teaspoons baking powder
½ teaspoon salt
¼ cup oil
1 cup water

Cycle: Quick bread or cake cycle. Add ingredients to the pan as described and assist the mixing as directed in the standard mixing instructions for quick breads on page 123.

Nutritional analysis per serving: 80 cal, 2.3 g protein, 12 g carbohydrate, 2.8 g fat, 0 g sat fat, 0 mg cholesterol, 111 mg sodium, 0.3 g fiber
   Serving size: approximately 1.0 ounce
   Servings per loaf: 21
   Diabetic exchanges: 1 starch/bread per serving

No-Yeast Whole Wheat Bread

Ingredients:

3 cups regular (not bread) whole wheat flour
3 teaspoons baking powder
½ teaspoon salt
¼ cup oil
1¼ cups water

Cycle: Quick bread or cake cycle. Add ingredients to the pan as described and assist the mixing as directed in the standard mixing instructions for quick breads on page 123.

Nutritional analysis per serving: 80 cal, 2.2 g protein, 12 g carbohydrate, 2.6 g fat, 0 g sat fat, 0 mg cholesterol, 97 mg sodium, 0.4 g fiber
  Serving size: approximately 1.0 ounce
  Servings per loaf: 24
  Diabetic exchanges: 1 starch/bread per serving

No-Yeast Whole Spelt Bread

Ingredients:

3 cups whole grain spelt flour
3 teaspoons baking powder
½ teaspoon salt
¼ cup oil
1¼ cups water

Cycle: Quick bread or cake cycle. Add ingredients to the pan as described and assist the mixing as directed in the standard mixing instructions for quick breads on page 123.

Nutritional analysis per serving: 80 cal, 2.2 g protein, 11.4 g carbohydrate, 2.8 g fat, 0 g sat fat, 0 mg cholesterol, 106 mg sodium, 1.1 g fiber
  Serving size: approximately 1.0 ounce
  Servings per loaf: 22
  Diabetic exchanges: 1 starch/bread per serving

No-Yeast Rye Bread

Ingredients:

   3 cups rye flour
   3 teaspoons baking powder
   ¾ teaspoon salt
   2 teaspoons caraway seed (optional)
   ⅓ cup oil
   1¼ cups water

Cycle: Quick bread or cake cycle. Add ingredients to the pan as described and assist the mixing as directed in the standard mixing instructions for quick breads on page 123.

Nutritional analysis per serving: 83 cal, 1.8 g protein, 12 g carbohydrate, 3.2 g fat, 0 g sat fat, 0 mg
        cholesterol, 118 mg sodium, 2 g fiber
   Serving size: approximately 1.0 ounce
   Servings per loaf: 24
   Diabetic exchanges: 1 starch/bread per serving

No-Yeast White Rye Bread

Ingredients:

   3 cups white rye flour (See "Sources," page 211)
   3 teaspoons baking powder
   ¾ teaspoon salt
   ⅓ cup oil
   1¼ cups water

Cycle: Quick bread or cake cycle. Add ingredients to the pan as described and assist the mixing as directed in the standard mixing instructions for quick breads on page 123.

Nutritional analysis per serving: 83 cal, 1.8 g protein, 12 g carbohydrate, 3.2 g fat, 0 g sat fat, 0 mg
        cholesterol, 118 mg sodium, 0.06 g fiber
   Serving size: approximately 1.0 ounce
   Servings per loaf: 24
   Diabetic exchanges: 1 starch/bread per serving

No-Yeast Barley Bread

Ingredients:

3 cups barley flour
3 teaspoons baking powder
¾ teaspoon salt
¼ cup oil
1¼ cups water

Cycle: Quick bread or cake cycle. Add ingredients to the pan as described and assist the mixing as directed in the standard mixing instructions for quick breads on page 123.

Nutritional analysis per serving: 82 cal, 1.4 g protein, 13 g carbohydrate, 2.5 g fat, 0 g sat fat, 0 mg cholesterol, 129 mg sodium, 0.08 g fiber
Serving size: approximately 1.0 ounce
Servings per loaf: 22
Diabetic exchanges: 1 starch/bread per serving

No-Yeast Kamut Bread

Ingredients:

3 cups kamut flour
3 teaspoon baking powder
¾ teaspoon salt
⅓ cup oil
1⅓ cups water

Cycle: Quick bread or cake cycle. Add ingredients to the pan as described and assist the mixing as directed in the standard mixing instructions for quick breads on page 123.

Nutritional analysis per serving: 82 cal, 1.8 g protein, 12 g carbohydrate, 3.1 g fat, 0 g sat fat, 0 mg cholesterol, 117 mg sodium, 2 g fiber
Serving size: approximately 1.1 ounce
Servings per loaf: 24
Diabetic exchanges: 1 starch/bread per serving

No-Yeast Gluten-Free Rice Bread

Ingredients:

1⅓ cup brown rice flour OR white rice flour

⅓ cup tapioca flour

⅓ cup potato flour

2¾ teaspoons guar gum

2¾ teaspoons baking powder

¾ teaspoon salt

1 tablespoon plus 1 teaspoon oil

2 extra large eggs OR ½ cup egg substitute

1⅓ cup water

Cycle: Quick bread or cake cycle. Add ingredients to the pan as described and assist the mixing as directed in the standard mixing instructions for quick breads on page 123.

Nutritional analysis per serving if made with eggs: 83 cal, 1.9 g protein, 14 g carbohydrate, 1.1 g fat, 0.3 g sat fat,43 mg cholesterol, 180 mg sodium, 0.4 g fiber with white rice flour, 0.8 g fiber with brown rice flour

Nutritional analysis per serving if made with egg substitute: 79 cal, 1.9 g protein, 14 g carbohydrate, 1.4 g fat, 0 g sat fat, 0 mg cholesterol, 184 mg sodium, 0.4 g fiber with white rice flour, 0.8 g fiber with brown rice flour

Serving size: approximately 1.4 ounce

Servings per loaf: 16

Diabetic exchanges: 1 starch/bread per serving

Corn Bread

Ingredients:

1½ cups all-purpose flour

½ cup cornmeal

2½ teaspoons baking powder

½ teaspoon salt

2 tablespoons oil

1 extra large egg OR ¼ cup egg substitute
    OR ¼ cup water in addition to the amount below

¼ cup Fruit Sweet™ or honey

⅜ cup water

Cycle: Quick bread or cake cycle. Add ingredients to the pan as described and assist the mixing as directed in the standard mixing instructions for quick breads on page 123.

Nutritional analysis per serving if made with egg: 79 cal, 1.8 g protein, 12.4 g carbohydrate, 2.3 g fat, 0.1 g sat fat, 21 mg cholesterol, 137 mg sodium, 0.05 g fiber
Nutritional analysis per serving if made with egg substitute: 77 cal, 1.8 g protein, 12.4 g carbohydrate, 2.5 g fat, 0 g sat fat, 0 mg cholesterol, 138 mg sodium, 0.05 g fiber
Nutritional analysis per serving if made with water: 72 cal, 1.3 g protein, 12.4 g carbohydrate, 1.9 g fat, 0 g sat fat, 0 mg cholesterol, 131 mg sodium, 0.05 g fiber
    Serving size: approximately 1.0 ounce
    Servings per loaf: 16
    Diabetic exchanges: 1 starch/bread per serving

Gluten-Free Corn Bread

Ingredients:

1 cup brown rice flour

½ cup cornmeal

⅓ cup tapioca flour

⅓ cup potato flour

3 teaspoons guar gum

3 teaspoons baking powder

½ teaspoon salt

2 tablespoons oil

2 extra large eggs OR ½ cup egg substitute

¼ cup Fruit Sweet™ or honey

⅝ cup water

Cycle: Quick bread or cake cycle. Add ingredients to the pan as described and assist the mixing as directed in the standard mixing instructions for quick breads on page 123.

Nutritional analysis per serving if made with eggs: 79 cal, 1.8 g protein, 12 g carbohydrate, 2 g fat, 0.2 g sat fat, 17 mg cholesterol, 125 mg sodium, 0.6 g fiber
Nutritional analysis per serving if made with egg substitute: 76 cal, 1.8 g protein, 12 g carbohydrate, 3 g fat, 0 g sat fat, 0 mg cholesterol, 127 mg sodium, 0.6 g fiber
    Serving size: approximately 1.1 ounce
    Servings per loaf: 20
    Diabetic exchanges: 1 starch/bread per serving

Wheat-Free Corn Bread

Ingredients:

1¾ cups white spelt flour
½ cup cornmeal
2½ teaspoons baking powder
½ teaspoon salt
2 tablespoons oil
1 extra large egg OR ¼ cup egg substitute
    OR ¼ cup water in addition to the amount below
¼ cup Fruit Sweet™ or honey
⅜ cup water

Cycle: Quick bread or cake cycle. Add ingredients to the pan as described and assist the mixing as directed in the standard mixing instructions for quick breads on page 123.

Nutritional analysis per serving if made with egg: 81 cal, 2.4 g protein, 13 g carbohydrate, 2.2 g fat, 0.1 g sat fat, 20 mg cholesterol, 129 mg sodium, 0.2 g fiber
Nutritional analysis per serving if made with egg substitute: 79 cal, 2.4 g protein, 13 g carbohydrate, 2.4 g fat, 0 g sat fat, 0 mg cholesterol, 130 mg sodium, 0.2 g fiber
Nutritional analysis per serving if made with water: 76 cal, 1.9 g protein, 13 g carbohydrate, 1.8 g fat, 0 g sat fat, 0 mg cholesterol, 124 mg sodium, 0.2 g fiber
    Serving size: approximately 1.0 ounce
    Servings per loaf: 17
    Diabetic exchanges: 1 starch/bread per serving

Applesauce Bread

Ingredients:

2 cups all-purpose flour
1 teaspoon baking powder
½ teaspoon baking soda
½ teaspoon salt (optional)
1 teaspoon cinnamon
¼ cup oil
½ cup unsweetened apple juice concentrate, thawed
¾ cup unsweetened applesauce
½ cup raisins (optional)

Cycle: Quick bread or cake cycle. Add ingredients to the pan as described and assist the mixing as directed in the standard mixing instructions for quick breads on page 123. Add the raisins after the liquids are thoroughly mixed in.

Nutritional analysis per serving without the raisins: 79 cal, 1.1 g protein, 12 g carbohydrate, 2.5 g fat, 0 g sat fat, 0 mg cholesterol, 53 mg sodium, 0.45 g fiber
Nutritional analysis per serving with the raisins: 90 cal, 1.1 g protein, 15 g carbohydrate, 2.5 g fat, 0 g sat fat, 0 mg cholesterol, 53 mg sodium, 0.15 g fiber
    Serving size: approximately 1.1 ounce
    Servings per loaf: 20
    Diabetic exchanges: 1 starch/bread per serving

Wheat-Free Applesauce Bread

Ingredients:

2⅜ cups white spelt flour

1 teaspoon baking powder

½ teaspoon baking soda

½ teaspoon salt (optional)

1 teaspoon cinnamon

¼ cup oil

½ cup unsweetened apple juice concentrate, thawed

¾ cup unsweetened applesauce

½ cup raisins (optional)

Cycle: Quick bread or cake cycle. Add ingredients to the pan as described and assist the mixing as directed in the standard mixing instructions for quick breads on page 123. Add the raisins after the liquids are thoroughly mixed in.

Nutritional analysis per serving without the raisins: 80 cal, 1.7 g protein, 12 g carbohydrate, 2.6 g fat, 0 g sat fat, 0 mg cholesterol, 89 mg sodium, 0.4 g fiber
Nutritional analysis per serving with the raisins: 91 cal, 1.8 g protein, 15 g carbohydrate, 2.6 g fat, 0 g sat fat, 0 mg cholesterol, 89 mg sodium, 0.7 g fiber
    Serving size: approximately 1.0 ounce
    Servings per loaf: 22
    Diabetic exchanges: 1 starch/bread per serving

Quinoa Applesauce Bread

Ingredients:

2½ cups quinoa flour
¾ cup tapioca flour
3 teaspoons baking powder
½ teaspoon baking soda
2 teaspoon cinnamon
¼ cup oil
¾ cup unsweetened apple juice concentrate, thawed
¾ cup unsweetened applesauce
½ cup raisins (optional)

Cycle: Quick bread or cake cycle. Add ingredients to the pan as described and assist the mixing as directed in the standard mixing instructions for quick breads on page 123. Add the raisins after the liquids are thoroughly mixed in.

Nutritional analysis per serving without the raisins: 79 cal, 1.1 g protein, 13.7 g carbohydrate, 2.2 g fat, 0 g sat fat, 0 mg cholesterol, 64 mg sodium, 0.5 g fiber
Nutritional analysis per serving with the raisins: 86 cal, 1.2 g protein, 15.6 g carbohydrate, 2.2 g fat, 0 g sat fat, 0 mg cholesterol, 64 mg sodium, 0.7 g fiber
Serving size: approximately 1.0 ounce
Servings per loaf: 29
Diabetic exchanges: 1 starch/bread per serving

Golden Fruit Bread

Ingredients:

3 cups kamut flour
3 teaspoons baking powder
¼ teaspoon salt
⅓ cup oil
1⅓ cup apple juice concentrate, thawed
⅓ cup dried blueberries, raisins, dried apricots cut into small pieces,
    or small pieces of the dried fruit of your choice

Cycle: Quick bread or cake cycle. Add ingredients to the pan as described and assist the mixing as directed in the standard mixing instructions for quick breads on page 123. Add the dried fruit after the apple juice is thoroughly mixed in. Watch the bread as the cycle nears completion, and if the sides of the loaf are getting too brown, test the bread for doneness by inserting a toothpick into the center of the bread. If the toothpick comes out dry, stop the cycle early and remove the bread from the machine.

Nutritional analysis per serving: 108 cal, 1.8 g protein, 19 g carbohydrate, 3 g fat, 0 g sat fat, 0 mg cholesterol, 77 mg sodium, 2.1 g fiber
Serving size: approximately 1.25 ounce
Servings per loaf: 25
Diabetic exchanges: 1 starch/bread + ½ fruit per serving

Date Nut Bread

Ingredients:

    2 cups all purpose flour
    ½ cup date sugar
    3 teaspoons baking powder
    ⅜ cup oil
    ¾ cup apple juice concentrate, thawed
    ¾ cup chopped dates
    ¾ cup chopped walnuts or other nuts

Cycle: Quick bread or cake cycle. Add ingredients to the pan as described and assist the mixing as directed in the standard mixing instructions for quick breads on page 123. Add the dates and nuts after the liquids are thoroughly mixed in. If the sides of this bread seem to be getting too brown before the baking time is up, test the center of the cake by inserting a toothpick into it. If it comes out dry, stop the cycle early and remove the bread.

Nutritional analysis per serving: 175 cal, 2.5 g protein, 26.5 g carbohydrate, 5.4 g fat, 0 g sat fat, 0 mg cholesterol, 77 mg sodium, 0.9 g fiber
Serving size: approximately 1.4 ounce
Servings per loaf: 18
Diabetic exchanges: 1 starch/bread + 1 fruit + 1 fat per serving

Spelt Date Nut Bread

Ingredients:

2¼ cups whole spelt or white spelt flour
½ cup date sugar
3 teaspoons baking powder
⅜ cup oil
¾ cup apple juice concentrate, thawed
¾ cup chopped dates
¾ cup chopped walnuts or other nuts

Cycle: Quick bread or cake cycle. Add ingredients to the pan as described and assist the mixing as directed in the standard mixing instructions for quick breads on page 123. Add the dates and nuts after the liquids are thoroughly mixed in. If the sides of this bread seem to be getting too brown before the baking time is up, test the center of the cake by inserting a toothpick into it. If it comes out dry, stop the cycle early and remove the bread.

Nutritional analysis per serving: 182 cal, 3.2 g protein, 28 g carbohydrate, 5.5 g fat, 0 g sat fat, 0 mg cholesterol, 77 mg sodium, 1.7 g fiber with whole spelt, 0.9 g fiber with white spelt
Serving size: approximately 1.4 ounce
Servings per loaf: 18
Diabetic exchanges: 1 starch/bread + 1 fruit + 1 fat per serving

Barley Date Nut Bread

Ingredients:

2 cups barley flour
½ cup date sugar
3 teaspoons baking powder
⅜ cup oil
¾ cup apple juice concentrate, thawed
¾ cup chopped dates
¾ cup chopped walnuts or other nuts

Cycle: Quick bread or cake cycle. Add ingredients to the pan as described and assist the mixing as directed in the standard mixing instructions for quick breads on page 123. Add the dates and nuts after the liquids are thoroughly mixed in. If the sides of this bread seem to be getting too brown before the baking time is up, test the center of the cake by inserting a toothpick into it. If it comes out dry, stop the cycle early and remove the bread.

Nutritional analysis per serving: 179 cal, 2.3 g protein, 28 g carbohydrate, 5.4 g fat, 0 g sat fat, 0 mg cholesterol, 77 mg sodium, 0.8 g fiber
　Serving size: approximately 1.4 ounce
　Servings per loaf: 18
　Diabetic exchanges: 1 starch/bread + 1 fruit + 1 fat per serving

Wheat-Free Banana Spice Cake

Ingredients:

2 cups barley flour

½ cup date sugar

3 teaspoons baking powder

1½ teaspoons cinnamon

¼ teaspoon cloves

¼ teaspoon allspice

¼ cup oil

2¼ cups pureed or thoroughly mashed bananas

½ teaspoon vanilla (optional)

Cycle: Quick bread or cake cycle. Add ingredients to the pan as described and assist the mixing as directed in the standard mixing instructions for quick breads on page 123. If the sides of this cake seem to be getting too brown before the baking time is up, test the center of the cake by inserting a toothpick into it. If it comes out dry, stop the cycle early and remove the cake.

Nutritional analysis per serving: 139 cal, 1.6 g protein, 28 g carbohydrate, 2.9 g fat, 0 g sat fat, 0 mg cholesterol, 66 mg sodium, 0.7 g fiber
　Serving size: approximately 1.5 ounce
　Servings per loaf: 20
　Diabetic exchanges: 1 starch/bread + l fruit per serving

Banana Spice Cake

Ingredients:

2 cups all purpose flour
½ cup date sugar
2½ teaspoons baking powder
½ teaspoon salt
1½ teaspoons cinnamon
¼ teaspoon cloves
¼ teaspoon allspice
¼ cup oil
2 cups pureed or thoroughly mashed bananas
½ teaspoon vanilla (optional)

Cycle: Quick bread or cake cycle. Add ingredients to the pan as described and assist the mixing as directed in the standard mixing instructions for quick breads on page 123.

Nutritional analysis per serving: 143 cal, 1.9 g protein, 28 g carbohydrate, 32 g fat, 0 g sat fat, 0 mg cholesterol, 117 mg sodium, 0.7 g fiber
Serving size: approximately 1.5 ounce
Servings per loaf: 18
Diabetic exchanges: 1 starch/bread + I fruit per serving

Gluten-Free Banana Spice Cake

Ingredients:

2¼ cups brown rice flour
½ cup tapioca flour
½ cup date sugar
3 teaspoons baking powder
1½ teaspoons cinnamon
¼ teaspoon cloves
¼ teaspoon allspice
¼ cup oil
2¼ cups pureed or thoroughly mashed bananas
½ teaspoons vanilla (optional)

Cycle: Quick bread or cake cycle. Add ingredients to the pan as described and assist the mixing as directed in the standard mixing instructions for quick breads on page 123. If the sides of this cake seem to be getting too brown before the baking time is up, test the center of the cake by inserting a toothpick into it. If it comes out dry, stop the cycle early and remove the cake.

Nutritional analysis per serving: 140 cal, 1.7 g protein, 29 g carbohydrate, 2.6 g fat, 0 g sat fat, 0 mg cholesterol, 57 mg sodium, 1 g fiber
    Serving size: approximately 1.5 ounce
    Servings per loaf: 23
    Diabetic exchanges: 1 starch/bread + I fruit per serving

Extra Nutrition Carrot Cake

Ingredients:

2⅛ cups whole wheat flour

1½ teaspoons baking soda

1 teaspoon cinnamon

¼ teaspoon cloves

3 tablespoons oil

⅔ cup pineapple juice concentrate

⅔ cup water

1 cup shredded carrots

½ cup raisins

Cycle: Quick bread or cake cycle. Add ingredients to the pan as described and assist the mixing as directed in the standard mixing instructions for quick breads on page 123. Add the carrots and raisins after the liquids are thoroughly mixed in.

Nutritional analysis per serving: 110 cal, 2.4 g protein, 20 g carbohydrate, 2.6 g fat, 0 g sat fat, 0 mg cholesterol, 86 mg sodium, 0.8 g fiber
    Serving size: approximately 1.4 ounce
    Servings per loaf: 18
    Diabetic exchanges: 1 starch/bread + ½ fruit per serving

Wheat-Free Extra Nutrition Carrot Cake

Ingredients:

2⅛ cups rye flour
1½ teaspoons baking soda
1 teaspoon cinnamon
¼ teaspoon cloves
3 tablespoons oil
⅔ cup pineapple juice concentrate
⅔ cup water
1 cup shredded carrots
½ cup raisins

Cycle: Quick bread or cake cycle. Add ingredients to the pan as described and assist the mixing as directed in the standard mixing instructions for quick breads on page 123. Add the carrots and raisins after the liquids are thoroughly mixed in.

Nutritional analysis per serving: 112 cal, 2.2 g protein, 21 g carbohydrate, 2.6 g fat, 0 g sat fat, 0 mg
cholesterol, 91 mg sodium, 1 g fiber
Serving size: approximately 1.4 ounce
Servings per loaf: 17
Diabetic exchanges: 1 starch/bread + ½ fruit per serving

Extra Nutrition Gingerbread

Ingredients:

2 cups whole wheat flour
2 teaspoons baking powder
1 teaspoon cinnamon
½ teaspoon ginger
3 tablespoons oil
½ cup molasses
½ cup water

Cycle: Quick bread or cake cycle. Add ingredients to the pan as described and assist the mixing as directed in the standard mixing instructions for quick breads on page 123.

Nutritional analysis per serving: 81 cal, 1.8 g protein, 14 g carbohydrate, 2.3 g fat, 0 g sat fat, 0 mg cholesterol, 52 mg sodium, 0.3 g fiber
Serving size: approximately 0.9 ounce
Servings per loaf: 20
Diabetic exchanges: 1 starch/bread per serving

Gluten-Free Chocolate Cake

Ingredients:

1¼ cups brown rice flour OR white rice flour

⅓ cup tapioca flour

⅓ cup potato flour

⅓ cup cocoa

2¾ teaspoons guar gum

2½ teaspoons baking powder + ½ teaspoon baking soda with Fruit Sweet™
OR 3 teaspoons baking powder with honey

¼ teaspoon salt

2 tablespoons oil

2 extra large eggs OR ½ cup egg substitute

¾ cup Fruit Sweet™ or honey

½ cup water

Cycle: Quick bread or cake cycle. Add ingredients to the pan as described and assist the mixing as directed in the standard mixing instructions for quick breads on page 123. If the sides of this cake seem to be getting too brown before the baking time is up, test the center of the cake by inserting a toothpick into it. If it comes out dry, stop the cycle early and remove the cake.

Nutritional analysis per serving if made with eggs: 110 cal, 1.9 g protein, 20 g carbohydrate, 2.4 g fat, 0.2 g sat fat, 34 mg cholesterol, 102 mg sodium, 0.7 g fiber with brown rice, 0.4 with white rice
Nutritional analysis per serving if made with egg substitute: 106 cal, 1.9 g protein, 20 g carbohydrate, 2.7g fat, 0.1 g sat fat, 0 mg cholesterol, 104 mg sodium, 0.7 g fiber with brown rice, 0.4 with white rice
Serving size: approximately 1.25 ounce
Servings per loaf: 20
Diabetic exchanges: 1 starch/bread + ½ fruit per serving

Wheat-Free Extra Nutrition Gingerbread

Ingredients:

2⅜ cups whole spelt flour

2 teaspoons baking powder

1 teaspoon cinnamon

½ teaspoon ginger

3 tablespoons oil

½ cup molasses

½ cup water

Cycle: Quick bread or cake cycle. Add ingredients to the pan as described and assist the mixing as directed in the standard mixing instructions for quick breads on page 123.

Nutritional analysis per serving: 79 cal, 1.7 g protein, 13 g carbohydrate, 2.1 g fat, 0 g sat fat, 0 mg
    cholesterol, 47 mg sodium, 0.9 g fiber
Serving size: approximately 0.9 ounce
Servings per loaf: 22
Diabetic exchanges: 1 starch/bread per serving

Chocolate Cake

Ingredients:

2⅓ cups all purpose flour

⅓ cup cocoa

3 teaspoons baking powder

¼ teaspoon salt

¼ cup oil

1¼ cups apple juice concentrate, thawed

Cycle: Quick bread or cake cycle. Add ingredients to the pan as described and assist the mixing as directed in the standard mixing instructions for quick breads on page 123. If the sides of this cake seem to be getting too brown before the baking time is up, test the center of the cake by inserting a toothpick into it. If it comes out dry, stop the cycle early and remove the cake.

Nutritional analysis per serving: 108 cal, 1.7 g protein, 18 g carbohydrate, 2.7 g fat, 0.1 g sat fat, 0 mg cholesterol, 101 mg sodium, 0.1 g fiber
    Serving size: approximately 1.2 ounce
    Servings per loaf: 19
    Diabetic exchanges: 1 starch/bread + ½ fruit per serving

Wheat-Free Chocolate Cake

Ingredients:

2¾ cups white spelt flour

⅓ cup cocoa

3 tsp. baking powder

¼ teaspoon salt

¼ cup oil

1¼ cups apple juice concentrate, thawed

Cycle: Quick bread or cake cycle. Add ingredients to the pan as described and assist the mixing as directed in the standard mixing instructions for quick breads on page 123. If the sides of this cake seem to be getting too brown before the baking time is up, test the center of the cake by inserting a toothpick into it. If it comes out dry, stop the cycle early and remove the cake.

Nutritional analysis per serving: 108 cal, 2.3 g protein, 18 g carbohydrate, 3 g fat, 0.1 g sat fat, 0 mg cholesterol, 101 mg sodium, 1.1 g fiber
    Serving size: approximately 1.2 ounce
    Servings per loaf: 21
    Diabetic exchanges: 1 starch/bread + ½ fruit per serving

Creamy Cake Topping

This sugar-free topping is great on chocolate cake, carrot cake, or gingerbread.

Ingredients:

½ cup unsalted cashews, macadamias, or shelled pine nuts
1 tablespoon tapioca flour
2 teaspoons cocoa (optional - use if you want chocolate topping)
⅓ cup Fruit Sweet™
½ teaspoon vanilla (optional)

Put the nuts and tapioca flour in a blender or food processor and process until the nuts are finely ground. Add the optional cocoa, if desired, and process for a few seconds. With the blender or processor running, slowly add the sweetener. Add the vanilla and process a few more seconds.

Nutritional analysis for the whole batch: To the whole batch values for the cake you are using, add 613 calories, 13 g. protein, 67 g. carbohydrate, 32 g. fat, 10 mg. sodium, and 6 g. fiber
Diabetic exchanges for the whole batch: 5 fruit + 7 fat

Heart Healthy Date Frosting

This fat-free, sugar-free frosting is good on banana spice cake or date nut bread.

Ingredients:

⅜ cup +1 tablespoon water
1 tablespoon all purpose flour OR 1 tablespoon white spelt flour
        OR 1 tablespoon barley flour OR 1 tablespoon + 1 teaspoon rice flour
⅔ cup date sugar

Combine the flour and water in a small saucepan. Bring them to a boil, reduce the heat, and simmer, stirring often, until the mixture is thick. Remove from the heat. Press the date sugar through a sieve to remove lumps. Add it to the flour mixture and beat until smooth. Frost the cake immediately before the frosting has time to cool.

Nutritional analysis for the whole batch: To the whole batch values for the cake you are using, add 428 calories, 107 g. carbohydrate, and 10 g. fiber
Diabetic exchanges for the whole batch: 7 fruit

Tortillas

People on special diets often long for more variety in what they eat. The recipes in this chapter and in the "Tortilla-Based Main Dishes and More" chapter on pages 161 to 173 will add some excitement to your diet.

Tortillas are easy to make using an electric tortilla maker. If you wish to make them by hand, follow the instructions on pages 16 to 17. This chapter provides recipes for fifteen types of tortillas made with a wide variety of flours. If you have food allergies, you will hopefully find several selections here that you can eat. If you need a few more "exotic ingredient" choices, see the tortillas recipes in *The Ultimate Food Allergy Cookbook and Survival Guide* as described on the last pages of this book. All of the recipes in this chapter will also be a welcome addition to low yeast or yeast-free diets.

Wheat and spelt contain a large amount of gluten which is ideal for making yeast breads but can cause problems when making tortillas. You must be careful not to over-mix or over-knead the tortilla dough or you may develop the gluten, resulting in rubbery tortillas. The oil in the wheat and spelt recipes also helps to produce tortillas that are tender.

STANDARD DIRECTIONS FOR WHEAT AND SPELT TORTILLAS: Begin heating your electric tortilla maker. Stir together the first (smaller) amount of flour listed in the recipe and the salt in a mixing bowl. Combine the water and oil and stir them together. Immediately stir them into the flour mixture to form a soft dough. Mix the dough BRIEFLY with your hands in the bowl or on a floured board, incorporating enough of the additional flour make the dough not sticky. Divide the dough into portions about the size of a small plum and shape them into balls. Let the dough for flour tortillas rest for one-half hour.

When the light goes off on the iron (indicating the end of the pre-heat cycle) slightly flatten one ball of dough and put it in the iron off-center toward the hinge. Close the press firmly and then release the pressure. With wheat or spelt tortillas, if you are not satisfied with the size of the tortilla, you can carefully press it again. Open the press and cook the tortilla for about one to two minutes. (It is all right if any blisters on the surface begin to brown. Then turn it with a non-stick spatula and cook the second side for about one minute more or until any blisters on the second also begins to brown.

STANDARD DIRECTIONS FOR LOWER GLUTEN TORTILLAS: Begin heating your electric tortilla maker. Put the flour, oats (if used), and salt (if used) in a bowl. Stir in the water and oil (if used). Mix the dough with a spoon until it is well mixed or, if necessary, use your hands. If needed, add an additional one to two tablespoons of water to make dough of a consistency slightly softer than Play-doh™. Divide the dough into portions about the size of a small plum and roll them into balls about 1½ inches in diameter.

When the light goes off on the iron (indicating the end of the pre-heat cycle) slightly flatten one ball of dough and put it in the iron off-center toward the hinge. Close the press firmly in one motion and then immediately release the pressure. After making a few tortillas you will know how hard to press to get a tortilla about 6 to 7 inches in diameter. (If you press too hard, the edges of the tortillas may become lacey).

Open the press and cook the tortilla for one to two minutes or until the edges begin to look dry. Then turn it with a non-stick spatula and cook the second side for about one to two minutes more. The tortilla should be set but not dry when it has been sufficiently cooked. If necessary, cook it longer, 30 seconds on each side. Some lower gluten tortillas may also develop blisters on the second side which may brown a little.

Some of these tortillas will be too fragile to roll around fillings. Simply serve them flat topped with the fillings of your choice or use them to make "Enchilada Casserole, page 167.

Flour Tortillas

Ingredients:

3¼ to 3½ cups all purpose or unbleached flour
1 teaspoon salt
⅓ cup oil
1 cup water

Prepare the dough and cook these tortillas following the standard directions for wheat and spelt tortillas on page 143 and the instruction booklet for your tortilla maker or the directions for cooking them by hand on pages 16 to 17.

Nutritional analysis per serving: 113 cal, 2.2 g protein, 16 g carbohydrate, 4 g fat, 0 g sat fat, 0 mg
cholesterol, 122 mg sodium, 0.6 g fiber
Serving size: 1 tortilla
Servings per batch: 19
Diabetic exchanges: 1 starch/bread, ¾ fat exchange per serving

White Spelt Tortillas

Ingredients:

3⅓ cups white spelt flour
¾ teaspoon salt
⅓ cup oil
½ cup water

Prepare the dough and cook these tortillas following the standard directions for wheat and spelt tortillas on page 143 and the instruction booklet for your tortilla maker or the directions for cooking them by hand on pages 16 to 17.

Nutritional analysis per serving: 111 cal, 2.9 g protein, 16 g carbohydrate, 4.5 g fat, 0 g sat fat, 0 mg cholesterol, 99 mg sodium, 0.7 g fiber
Serving size: 1 tortilla
Servings per batch: 18
Diabetic exchanges: 1 starch/bread, 0.9 fat exchange per serving

Whole Wheat Tortillas

Ingredients:

3 to 3¼ cups whole wheat flour
1 teaspoon salt
⅓ cup oil
1 cup water

Prepare the dough and cook these tortillas following the standard directions for wheat and spelt tortillas on page 143 and the instruction booklet for your tortilla maker or the directions for cooking them by hand on pages 16 to 17.

Nutritional analysis per serving: 115 cal, 3.1 g protein, 16 g carbohydrate, 4.8 g fat, 0 g sat fat, 0 mg cholesterol, 139 mg sodium, 2.8 g fiber
Serving size: 1 tortilla
Servings per batch: 17
Diabetic exchanges: 1 starch/bread, 0.9 fat exchange per serving

Whole Spelt Tortillas

Ingredients:

4¼ to 4½ cups whole spelt flour
1 teaspoon salt
½ cup oil
1¼ cups water

Prepare the dough and cook these tortillas following the standard directions for wheat and spelt tortillas on page 143 and the instruction booklet for your tortilla maker or the directions for cooking them by hand on pages 16 to 17.

Nutritional analysis per serving: 122 cal, 3.1 g protein, 18 g carbohydrate, 5.4 g fat, 0 g sat fat, 0 mg
cholesterol, 107 mg sodium, 3.9 g fiber
Serving size: 1 tortilla
Servings per batch: 22
Diabetic exchanges: 1 starch/bread, 1 fat exchange per serving

Corn Tortillas

Ingredients:

3 cups masa harina*
2 cups warm water

Prepare the dough and cook these tortillas following the standard directions for lower gluten tortillas on pages 143 to 144 and the instruction booklet for your tortilla maker or the directions for cooking them by hand on pages 16 to 17. Also, for corn tortillas, keep the tortilla dough or balls covered with plastic wrap as you are cooking the tortillas so that the dough does not dry out.

*Note: Masa harina is corn flour that has been specially prepared for making tortillas. If you cannot find it in your grocery store, see "Sources," page 212.

Nutritional analysis per serving: 78 cal, 2.0 g protein, 16 g carbohydrate, 0.8 g fat, 0 g sat fat, 0 mg
cholesterol, 1 mg sodium, 2.9 g fiber
Serving size: 1 tortilla
Servings per batch: 16
Diabetic exchanges: 1 starch/bread per serving

Kamut Tortillas

Ingredients:

4 cups kamut flour
1 teaspoon salt
1⅝ cups (1½ cups plus 2 tablespoons) water

Prepare the dough and cook these tortillas following the standard directions for lower gluten tortillas on pages 143 to 144 and the instruction booklet for your tortilla maker or the directions for cooking them by hand on pages 16 to 17. Kamut tortillas often have blisters which brown slightly on the side of the tortilla which you cook second.

Nutritional analysis per serving: 80 cal, 2.9 g protein, 18 g carbohydrate, 0.4 g fat, 0 g sat fat, 0 mg cholesterol, 107 mg sodium, 2.9 g fiber
Serving size: 1 tortilla
Servings per batch: 22
Diabetic exchanges: 1 starch/bread per serving

Rye Tortillas

Ingredients:

4 cups rye flour
1 teaspoon salt
1½ cups water

Prepare the dough and cook these tortillas following the standard directions for lower gluten tortillas on pages 143 to 144 and the instruction booklet for your tortilla maker or the directions for cooking them by hand on pages 16 to 17.

Nutritional analysis per serving: 80 cal, 2.1 g protein, 17.6 g carbohydrate, 0.4 g fat, 0 g sat fat, 0 mg cholesterol, 147 mg sodium, 3.7 g fiber
Serving size: 1 tortilla
Servings per batch: 18
Diabetic exchanges: 1 starch/bread per serving

Barley Tortillas

Ingredients:

4 cups barley flour
1 teaspoon salt
1⅛ cups (1 cup plus 2 tablespoons) water

Prepare the dough and cook these tortillas following the standard directions for lower gluten tortillas on pages 143 to 144 and the instruction booklet for your tortilla maker or the directions for cooking them by hand on pages 16 to 17.

Nutritional analysis per serving: 82 cal, 2.7 g protein, 17 g carbohydrate, 0.4 g fat, 0 g sat fat, 0 mg cholesterol, 130 mg sodium, 2.7 g fiber
Serving size: 1 tortilla
Servings per batch: 18
Diabetic exchanges: 1 starch/bread per serving

Buckwheat Tortillas

Ingredients:

4 cups buckwheat flour
1 teaspoon salt
1¾ cups water

Prepare the dough and cook these tortillas following the standard directions for lower gluten tortillas on pages 143 to 144 and the instruction booklet for your tortilla maker or the directions for cooking them by hand on pages 16 to 17.

Nutritional analysis per serving: 80 cal, 3.0 g protein, 17 g carbohydrate, 0.7 g fat, 0 g sat fat, 0 mg cholesterol, 120 mg sodium, 2.4 g fiber
Serving size: 1 tortilla
Servings per batch: 20
Diabetic exchanges: 1 starch/bread per serving

Garbanzo Tortillas

Ingredients:

4 cups garbanzo flour
1 teaspoon salt
1 cup water

Prepare the dough and cook these tortillas following the standard directions for lower gluten tortillas on pages 143 to 144 and the instruction booklet for your tortilla maker or the directions for cooking them by hand on pages 16 to 17.

Nutritional analysis per serving: 83 cal, 4.5 g protein, 14 g carbohydrate, 1.5 g fat, 0 g sat fat, 0 mg cholesterol, 156 mg sodium, 0.8 g fiber
Serving size: 1 tortilla
Servings per batch: 15
Diabetic exchanges: 1 starch/bread per serving

Teff Tortillas

Ingredients:

4 cups teff flour
1 teaspoon salt
1½ cups water

Prepare the dough and cook these tortillas following the standard directions for lower gluten tortillas on pages 143 to 144 and the instruction booklet for your tortilla maker or the directions for cooking them by hand on pages 16 to 17.

Nutritional analysis per serving: 79 cal, 2.6 g protein, 15.8 g carbohydrate, 0.6 g fat, 0 g sat fat, 0 mg cholesterol, 110 mg sodium, 3.0 g fiber
Serving size: 1 tortilla
Servings per batch: 22
Diabetic exchanges: 1 starch/bread per serving

Oat Tortillas

Ingredients:

3 cups oat flour
1 cup quick-cooking oats
1 teaspoon salt
1¼ cups water

Prepare the dough and cook these tortillas following the standard directions for lower gluten tortillas on pages 143 to 144 and the instruction booklet for your tortilla maker or the directions for cooking them by hand on pages 16 to 17.

Nutritional analysis per serving: 87 cal, 3.6 g protein, 15 g carbohydrate, 1.5 g fat, 0 g sat fat, 0 mg cholesterol, 147 mg sodium, 2.8 g fiber
Serving size: 1 tortilla
Servings per batch: 16
Diabetic exchanges: 1 starch/bread per serving

Rice Tortillas

Ingredients:

4 cups brown rice or white rice flour
1 teaspoon salt
2 tablespoons oil
2 cups water

Prepare the dough and cook these tortillas following the standard directions for lower gluten tortillas on pages 143 to 144 and the instruction booklet for your tortilla maker or the directions for cooking them by hand on pages 16 to 17.

Nutritional analysis per serving: 90 cal, 1.6 g protein, 17 g carbohydrate, 1.6 g fat, 0 g sat fat, 0 mg cholesterol, 86 mg sodium, 1.0 g fiber with brown rice flour, 0.6 g fiber with white rice flour
    Serving size: 1 tortilla
    Servings per batch: 28
    Diabetic exchanges: 1 starch/bread, 0.2 fat exchange per serving

Amaranth Tortillas

Ingredients:

4½ cups amaranth flour
1 teaspoon salt
1½ cups water

Prepare the dough and cook these tortillas following the standard directions for lower gluten tortillas on pages 143 to 144 and the instruction booklet for your tortilla maker or the directions for cooking them by hand on pages 16 to 17.

Nutritional analysis per serving: 82 cal, 3.0 g protein, 14.3 g carbohydrate, 1.1 g fat, 0 g sat fat, 0 mg cholesterol, 98 mg sodium, 1.5 g fiber
    Serving size: 1 tortilla
    Servings per batch: 24
    Diabetic exchanges: 1 starch/bread per serving

Quinoa Tortillas

Ingredients:

4 cups quinoa flour
1 teaspoon salt
1½ cups water

Prepare the dough and cook these tortillas following the standard directions for lower gluten tortillas on pages 143 to 144 and the instruction booklet for your tortilla maker or the directions for cooking them by hand on pages 16 to 17.

Nutritional analysis per serving: 79 cal, 2.8 g protein, 14.6 g carbohydrate, 1.2 g fat, 0 g sat fat, 0 mg cholesterol, 102 mg sodium, 1.3 g fiber
    Serving size: 1 tortilla
    Servings per batch: 24
    Diabetic exchanges: 1 starch/bread per serving

Bread-Based Main Dishes and Snacks

Dumpling Pie

Filling Ingredients:

½ cup chopped celery
¼ cup chopped onion OR additional chopped celery
2 tablespoons oil
3 tablespoons all purpose flour OR white spelt flour
¼ teaspoon dry sweet basil OR 1 teaspoon fresh chopped sweet basil
¼ teaspoon pepper
1½ cups chicken or turkey broth
1½ cups peas, frozen or fresh
2 cups cubed cooked turkey or chicken

To make the filling, sauté the celery and onion in the 2 tablespoons oil until they begin to brown. Add the 3 tablespoons flour and stir and cook 1 minute. Add the seasonings and broth; bring the mixture to a boil and cook a few minutes until it is thickened. Stir in the peas and chicken or turkey. Put the filling into a 2½ to 3-quart casserole dish. Preheat the oven to 400°F while mixing the topping ingredients.

Topping Ingredients:

1 cup all purpose OR white spelt flour
1 teaspoon baking powder
¼ teaspoon salt
¼ teaspoon dry sweet basil OR 1 teaspoon fresh chopped sweet basil
2 tablespoons oil
⅓ cup water

To make the topping, put the 1 cup flour, baking powder, salt, and basil into your bread machine pan. Set the cycle to "mix," cake," or "quick bread" (non-yeast) if your machine has any of those cycles; otherwise, hand-mixing (see pages 18 to 19) or the first few minutes of any cycle without a pre-heat will work fine. Start the machine and let it mix for ½ to 1 minute. (If it mixes very slowly at first, begin timing when the fast, continuous mixing begins). Add the oil and allow it to mix another minute. Add the water and allow the machine to mix for about 2 minutes, or until about 30 seconds after the dough has become a cohesive ball around the bread machine blade. Stop the machine.

Remove the dough from the machine and drop heaping teaspoonfuls of it onto the filling mixture in the casserole. Bake for 30 to 35 minutes, or until the dumplings are lightly browned.

Nutritional analysis per serving: 279 cal, 19 g protein, 23 g carbohydrate, 9 g fat, 0,8 g sat fat, 36 mg cholesterol, 331 mg sodium, 1.8 g fiber
Serving size: $\frac{1}{6}$ of the batch
Servings per batch: 6
Diabetic exchanges per serving: 2 starch/bread + 2 lean meat

Heart Healthy Burgers

Ingredients:

1 pound ground turkey
½ pound ground buffalo
1 cup cooked grain of any kind or combination
1 cup cooked vegetables, any kind or combination (peas, beans, and carrots are good)
1 teaspoon salt, or to taste (optional)
Hamburger buns, page 112

Briefly puree the grains and vegetables in a food processor or blender. (They do not have to be liquefied; a few chunks remaining in the burgers are nice). Combine the puree with the turkey, buffalo, and salt and form the mixture into 10 patties. Broil 5 to 8 minutes on each side and serve with the buns. These patties freeze well.

Nutritional analysis per serving: 140 cal, 19 g protein, 6 g carbohydrate, 3.7 g fat, 1.3 g sat fat, 50 mg cholesterol, 259 mg sodium, 0.3 g fiber
Serving size: approximately 3.0 ounces
Servings per batch: 10
Diabetic exchanges per serving: 2 lean meat + ½ starch/bread

Note: These nutritional values are based on using brown rice for the grain and ⅓ cup each of peas, carrots, and green beans. The values are for the burgers only and do not include the hamburger buns.

Tamale Pie

Filling Ingredients:

¼ cup chopped bell pepper (about ½ pepper)
½ small onion, chopped (optional)
1 tablespoon oil
1 15-ounce can tomatoes
1 teaspoon chili powder or to taste
1 4-ounce can sliced mushrooms, drained
1 14-ounce can black beans, drained
1 cup cubed cooked turkey or chicken

To make the filling, sauté the pepper and onion in the oil until they begin to brown. Coarsely chop the tomatoes and add them and their juice to the saucepan. Stir in the chili powder, mushrooms, beans, and chicken or turkey and bring the mixture to a boil. Pour it into a 2½ to 3-quart casserole dish. Preheat the oven to 350°F while mixing the topping.

Topping Ingredients:

½ cup all purpose OR white spelt flour
½ cup cornmeal
2 teaspoons baking powder
¼ teaspoon salt
2 tablespoons oil
½ cup water

To make the topping, put the flour, cornmeal, baking powder, and salt into your bread machine pan. Set the cycle to "mix," cake," or "quick bread" (non-yeast) if your machine has any of those cycles; otherwise, hand-mixing (see pages 18 to 19) or the first few minutes of any cycle without a pre-heat is fine. Start the machine and let it mix for ½ to 1 minute. (If it mixes very slowly at first, begin timing when the fast, continuous mixing begins). Add the oil and allow it to mix another minute. Add the water and allow the machine to mix for another 1 to 2 minutes. Stop the machine. Spread the batter over the filling mixture in the casserole dish. Bake for 30 to 35 minutes, or until the topping begins to brown.

Nutritional analysis per serving: 264 cal, 15 g protein, 31 g carbohydrate, 8.5 g fat, 0.3 g sat fat, 18 mg cholesterol, 670 mg sodium, 5 g fiber
Serving size: $\frac{1}{6}$ of the batch
Servings per batch: 6
Diabetic exchanges per serving: 2 starch/bread + 2 lean meat

Heart Healthy Pizza

Dough ingredients*:

¾ cup water
2½ tablespoons apple juice concentrate, thawed,
     OR 1½ tablespoon Fruit Sweet™ or honey plus 1 tablespoon water
1 tablespoon oil
½ teaspoon salt
2¼ cups bread flour
1¼ teaspoons active dry yeast

Sauce ingredients (for 2 pizzas - freeze half for future use):

1 6-ounce can tomato paste
1 8-ounce can tomato sauce
½ cup water
1 teaspoon dry oregano OR 1 tablespoon chopped fresh oregano
½ teaspoon dry thyme OR 1 teaspoon chopped fresh thyme
½ teaspoon dry sweet basil OR 1 teaspoon chopped fresh sweet basil

Topping ingredients:

2 to 3 ounces low fat or part-skim mozzarella cheese
2 tablespoons grated Romano cheese
½ cup chopped vegetables of your choice - green peppers, mushrooms, etc.
2 ounces cooked lean ground meat (optional)

Start the dough in your bread machine using the dough cycle. Combine the sauce ingredients in a saucepan, bring them to a boil, reduce the heat, and simmer them for 30 to 40 minutes, stirring occasionally. Grate the cheese and chop the vegetables. Preheat your oven to 400°F. When the dough cycle is finished, remove the dough from the bread machine and stretch it out in a lightly oiled 12-inch pizza pan. Spread it with half of the sauce and sprinkle it with the toppings. If you prefer "thick crust" pizza, allow the pizza to rise for 20 to 30 minutes. For a thinner crust, bake it as soon as you finish making it. Bake for 25 to 30 minutes, or until the edge of the pizza is brown.

*Note: For whole-wheat pizza, substitute a one-pound batch of dough made using the whole wheat bread recipes on pages 74 or 75 for the dough in this recipe.

Nutritional analysis per serving: 205 cal, 7 g protein, 27 g carbohydrate, 7 g fat, 1 g sat fat, 7 mg cholesterol, 367 mg sodium, 0.3 g fiber
Serving size: $\frac{1}{9}$ of the pizza
Servings per batch: 9 (or cut into 6 wedges and multiply the nutritional values by 1½)
Diabetic exchanges per serving: 2 starch/bread + ½ medium fat meat + ½ vegetable

Wheat-Free Heart Healthy Pizza

Dough ingredients*:

⅔ cup water
2½ tablespoons apple juice concentrate, thawed
1 tablespoon oil
½ teaspoon salt
2¼ cups white spelt flour
1¾ teaspoons active dry yeast

Sauce and topping ingredients: same as for "Heart Healthy Pizza," page 154

Put the dough ingredients into your bread machine and start the dough cycle. Make the sauce and top and bake the pizza as in "Heart Healthy Pizza," page 154.

*Note: For other varieties of wheat-free pizza, substitute a one-pound batch of dough made using the bread recipes on pages 76, bottom of 78, 81, or top of 84 or about ¾ of a batch of dough made using the recipes on pages 85 or top of 86 for the white spelt dough in this recipe. If you use a partial batch of dough for pizza, make the rest of the batch into rolls.

Nutritional analysis per serving: 209 cal, 8.5 g protein, 28 g carbohydrate, 7 g fat, 1 g sat fat, 7 mg cholesterol, 373 mg sodium, 0.7 g fiber
Serving size: $\frac{1}{9}$ of the pizza
Servings per batch: 9 (or cut into 6 wedges and multiply the nutritional values by 1½)
Diabetic exchanges per serving: 2 starch/bread + ½ medium fat meat + ½ vegetable

Gluten-Free Pizza

Ingredients:

1 1-pound batch of dough made with "Gluten-free Rice Potato Bread" recipe, page 76
   OR substitute about ¾ of a batch of dough made with the recipes for "Amaranth
   Bread," page 82, Buckwheat Bread, page 82, or Quinoa Bread, page 83

Sauce and topping ingredients: same as for "Heart Healthy Pizza," page 154

Put the bread ingredients into your bread machine and start the dough cycle. Make the
sauce and top and bake the pizza as in "Heart Healthy Pizza," page 154. If you use a partial
batch of bread dough, make the remaining dough into rolls.

Nutritional analysis per serving if made with rice potato bread dough with eggs: 192 cal, 8 g protein,
   25 g carbohydrate, 5.7 g fat, 1.4 g sat fat, 75 mg cholesterol, 457 mg sodium, 1.3 g fiber
Nutritional analysis per serving if made with rice potato bread dough with egg substitute: 192 cal, 8
   g protein, 25 g carbohydrate, 6.4 g fat, 1.0 g sat fat, 6 mg cholesterol, 515 mg sodium, 1.3 g fiber
Serving size: $\frac{1}{10}$ of the pizza
Servings per batch: 10 (or cut into 7 wedges and multiply the nutritional values by 1½)
Diabetic exchanges per serving: 2 starch/bread + ½ medium fat meat + ½ vegetable

Easy Vegetarian Burgers

Ingredients:

1 8-ounce can tomato sauce
¾ cup textured vegetable protein (dry flakes)
¾ cup oatmeal, uncooked
1 extra large egg OR ¼ cup egg substitute
½ teaspoon salt
¼ teaspoon pepper
1 tablespoon chopped fresh onion OR 1 teaspoon dry minced onion flakes (optional)
Hamburger buns, page 112

Bring the tomato sauce to a boil in a saucepan. Stir in the textured vegetable protein,
remove the pan from the heat, and allow it to stand for 5 to 10 minutes, or until the liquid is

all absorbed. Mix in the rest of the ingredients (except the buns). Form the mixture into 6 patties. Cook them in a lightly oiled or non-stick skillet until they brown lightly on both sides. These burgers freeze well, both before and after cooking.

Nutritional analysis (not including the bun) per serving if made with eggs: 101 cal, 11.5 g protein, 11 g carbohydrate, 1.8 g fat, 0.3 g sat fat, 57 mg cholesterol, 333 mg sodium, 0.1 g fiber
Nutritional analysis (not including the bun) per serving if made with egg substitute: 95 cal, 11.5 g protein, 11 g carbohydrate, 2.3 g fat, 0 g sat fat, 0 mg cholesterol, 389 mg sodium, 0.1 g fiber
Serving size: one burger
Servings per batch: 6
Diabetic exchanges per serving: 1 lean meat + ½ starch/bread

Calzones

Ingredients:

1 batch of dough from any of the following recipes:
Any 1½ pound batch of dough made with a basic bread recipe, pages 60 to 71
Any 1½ pound batch of dough made with a whole grain bread recipe, pages 73 to 78, 81, top of 84, bottom of 86 to 88, top of 90, or 92
¾ cup low fat or part-skim ricotta cheese
¼ cup grated Romano cheese
¼ pound low fat or part skim mozzarella cheese, coarsely grated
½ to ¾ cup pizza sauce, about ¼ of a batch of the sauce recipe on page 154

Cycle: Dough cycle, using the bread ingredients only. When the cycle is finished, divide the dough into 8 to 10 pieces and roll each piece out into a 6-inch to 7-inch circle on a lightly floured board. Mix the cheeses and put the mixture on the circles of dough, evenly dividing it between the circles of dough. Top each cheese portion with about 1 tablespoon of sauce. Moisten the edges of the circles with a small amount of water and fold the circles in half over the filling, crimping the edges together. Prick the tops of the calzones with a sharp knife. Transfer them to a lightly oiled baking sheet and allow to rise in a warm place for 15 to 20 minutes. Preheat the oven to 400°F. Bake the calzones for 20 to 25 minutes, or until brown.

Nutritional analysis per serving for filling only: 94 cal, 8 g protein, 2.6 g carb, 5.3 g fat, 3 g sat fat, 21 mg chol, 383 mg sodium, 0 g fiber (Add the nutritional values for $\frac{1}{10}$ batch of the bread used).
Serving size: 1 calzone
Servings per batch: 10
Diabetic exchanges per serving: 1 medium fat meat + $\frac{1}{3}$ vegetable + approximately 2 starch/bread for the dough. (Divide the number of starch/bread exchanges per batch of the bread recipe used by 10).

Mexican Strata

Ingredients:

3 to 4 slices of bread from any recipe in this book or commercially made bread
1 pound fresh or frozen corn
2 pounds zucchini or crookneck squash, thinly sliced
1 4-ounce can diced green chiles, drained
4 ounces low fat Monterey jack cheese, coarsely grated
3 eggs OR ¾ cup egg substitute
1¾ cups skim milk
½ teaspoon salt
⅛ teaspoon pepper

Cut and piece the bread to fit the bottom of an 11-inch by 7-inch baking dish. Spread the corn on top of the bread. Cover it with the squash. Spread the chiles on top of the squash. Sprinkle the whole dish with grated cheese. Beat together the remaining ingredients and pour them over the whole dish. Refrigerate overnight or a few hours if desired. Bake, uncovered, at 375°F for 30 to 40 minutes, or until it puffs up and begins to brown.

Nutritional analysis per serving if made with eggs: 192 cal, 13.5 g protein, 20 g carbohydrate, 8.7 g fat, 3 g sat fat, 195 mg cholesterol, 437 mg sodium, 2.3 g fiber
Nutritional analysis per serving: 191 cal, 13.5 g protein, 20 g carbohydrate, 10.1 g fat, 2 g sat fat, 13 mg cholesterol, 450 mg sodium, 2.3 g fiber
Serving size: ⅙ batch
Servings per batch: 6
Diabetic exchanges per serving: 1½ starch/bread + 1½ low fat meat

Breadsticks

Ingredients:

1 batch of dough from any of these recipes:
    Any 1½ pound batch of dough made with a basic bread recipe, pages 60 to 71
    Any 1½ pound batch of dough made with a whole grain bread recipe, pages 73 to 78, 81, bottom of 86 to 88, top of 90, or 92
    1 pound batch of Kamut Bread, page 84
1 lightly beaten egg white OR 1 batch of "Bread or Bun Wash," page 111
Optional for seeded breadsticks – ½ cup sesame seeds OR ¼ cup poppy seeds

Cycle: Dough cycle. When the cycle is finished, remove the dough from the machine and divide it into 18 or more pieces. On a lightly floured board, roll each piece into a 10-inch long rope. Place them on a lightly oiled baking sheet and brush them with the egg white or wash. Allow them to rise in a warm place for 30 minutes. Preheat your oven and bake at 375°F for 15 to 25 minutes, or until they are brown. Remove them from the baking sheet immediately and cool them on a wire rack. For seeded breadsticks, after rolling the dough into ropes, brush the breadsticks with the egg white or wash while they are still on the work surface. Then roll them in the seeds and transfer them to the baking sheet. Allow to rise and bake as above.

Nutritional Analysis: For plain breadsticks, divide the whole batch values for the bread recipe you used by the number of breadsticks you made. For sesame seed breadsticks, add 322 calories, 9.6 g protein, 15 g carbohydrate, 27 g fat, 6 mg sodium, and 11 g fiber to the whole batch bread values; then divide by the number of breadsticks made. For poppy seed breadsticks, add 190 calories, 6 g protein, 8 g carbohydrate, 16 g fat, 7 mg. sodium, and 3 g fiber to the whole batch bread values; then divide by the number of breadsticks made.

Diabetic exchanges per serving: Divide the number of starch/bread exchanges in a whole batch of the bread recipe you used by the number of breadsticks made.

Vegetable Calzones

Ingredients:

1 batch of dough from any of the following recipes:
> Any 1½ pound batch of dough made with a basic bread recipe, pages 60 to 71
> Any 1½ pound batch of dough made with a whole grain bread recipe, pages 73 to 78, 81, top of 84, bottom of 86 to 88, top of 90, or 92

2 to 3 cups cooked vegetables, any kind or combination, such as beans, carrots, small pieces of broccoli, sautéed mushrooms or onions

¼ pound low fat or part-skim mozzarella cheese, low fat cheddar cheese, or low fat Monterey jack cheese, coarsely grated

½ to ¾ cup pizza sauce, about ¼ of a batch of the sauce recipe on page 154 (optional)

Cycle: Dough cycle, using the bread ingredients only. When the cycle is finished, divide the dough into 8 to 10 pieces and roll each piece out into a 6-inch to 7-inch circle on a lightly floured board. Divide the vegetables evenly between the circles of dough. Top each with cheese. Top each cheese portion with about 1 tablespoon of sauce. Moisten the edges of the circles with a small amount of water and fold the circles in half over the filling, crimping the edges together. Prick the tops of the calzones with a sharp knife. Transfer them to a lightly oiled baking sheet and allow to rise in a warm place for 15 to 20 minutes. Preheat the oven to 400°F. Bake the calzones for 20 to 25 minutes, or until brown.

Nutritional analysis per serving for filling only: 52 cal, 4.6 g protein, 3.4 g carbohydrate, 2.5 g fat, 1.2 g sat fat, 8 mg cholesterol, 102 mg sodium, 1.2 g fiber (Add the nutritional values for $\frac{1}{10}$ batch of the bread used).
Serving size: 1 calzone
Servings per batch: 10
Diabetic exchanges per serving: ½ medium fat meat + ½ vegetable + approximately 2 starch/bread for the dough. (Divide the number of starch/bread exchanges per batch of the bread recipe used by 10).

Pretzels

Ingredients:

1 batch of dough from any of these recipes:
    Any 1½ pound batch of dough made with a basic bread recipe, pages 60 to 71
    Any 1½ pound batch of dough made with a whole grain bread recipe, pages 73 to
        78, 81, bottom of 86 to 88, top of 90, or 92
    1 pound batch of Kamut Bread, page 84
1 lightly beaten egg white OR 1 batch of "Bread or Bun Wash," page 111
1½ teaspoons coarse kosher salt

Cycle: Dough cycle. When the cycle is finished, remove the dough from the machine and divide it into 25 to 30 pieces. (One way to do this is to the roll the dough out ½ inch thick on a lightly floured board and cut it into strips). Lightly flour your hands and work surface, and roll each piece into a 12-inch to 15-inch long rope. Twist each rope into a pretzel or open knot shape. Place them on a lightly oiled baking sheet and brush them with the egg white or wash. Sprinkle them with the salt. Allow them to rise in a warm place for 30 minutes. Preheat your oven and bake at 350°F for 20 to 25 minutes, or until they are lightly brown. Remove them from the baking sheet immediately and cool them on a wire rack.

Nutritional Analysis: To the whole batch values for the bread recipe you used add 3000 mg sodium. Divide by the number of pretzels you made to get the values per pretzel.
Diabetic exchanges per serving: Divide the number of starch/bread exchanges in a whole batch of the bread recipe you used by the number of pretzels made.

Tortilla-Based Main Dishes and More

The recipes in this chapter will add some pizzazz to your life. If you are not allergic to wheat and corn, you can use commercially made tortillas to make the recipes in this chapter. You will find many good brands of additive-free wheat and corn tortillas at your grocery store, and health food stores carry spelt tortillas. (Or see "Sources," page 213).

The nutritional values for the recipes in this chapter are based on the values for wheat or corn tortillas. If you use a different kind of tortilla, the nutritional analysis will be similar and the diabetic exchanges should be about the same if you use the same size tortilla.

Be adventurous in your cooking and enjoy these new dishes!

Easy Burritos

Ingredients:

1½ pounds extra lean ground beef
2 cups bottled salsa or salsa fresca (recipe on page 170)
1 6-ounce can tomato paste
½ teaspoon chipotle powder (other chili powder may be substituted) or to taste
16 burrito-sized flour tortillas
2 to 3 15-ounce cans refried beans
16 ounces of shredded low-fat cheddar cheese

Cook the beef in a frying pan, stirring it and breaking it up, until it is brown throughout. Add the salsa, tomato paste, and chipotle or chili powder, and simmer the meat mixture for about 5 more minutes.

Spread about $\frac{1}{8}$ to $\frac{1}{6}$ can of the refried beans down the middle of each tortilla. Top the beans with $\frac{1}{16}$ of the beef-tomato mixture, and sprinkle with $\frac{1}{16}$ of the cheese. Fold over one side of the burrito, fold the ends in, and roll it up over the other side of the burrito. Use a toothpick to hold each burrito closed or put them on a dish seam-side down. You may wrap the burritos in plastic wrap and refrigerate or freeze them at this point. When you are ready to eat them, microwave each burrito for 2 to 3 minutes or until it is hot throughout.

Nutritional analysis per serving based on using flour (wheat) tortillas: 404 cal, 25 g protein, 53 g carbohydrate, 11.4 g fat, 4.0 g sat fat, 21 mg cholesterol, 873 mg sodium, 5.5 g fiber
Serving size: 1 burrito
Servings per batch: 16
Diabetic exchanges per serving: 3½ starch/bread + $1\frac{1}{8}$ very lean meat + 1¼ lean meat + 1 fat

Vegetarian Burritos

Ingredients:

> 1⅛ cup water
> ½ cup uncooked regular white rice (or substitute 1 cup cooked brown rice
>   or grain of your choice for the water and rice)
> ½ teaspoon garlic salt or salt
> 1 jalapeno pepper, or to taste
> 2 15-ounce cans black beans
> Shredded cheddar or Monterey jack cheese (optional)
> 10 to 15 flour, whole wheat, white spelt, or whole spelt tortillas*
> Optional additional filling ingredients for non-vegetarian burritos:
>   2 large tomatoes, diced, or ¾ cup salsa fresca or bottled salsa
>   2 cups shredded chicken (recipe on page 166)
> Optional toppings of your choice:
>   Shredded cheddar or Monterey jack cheese
>   Salsa, bottled or homemade salsa fresca (recipe on page 170)
>   Guacamole (recipe on page 171)

Put the water in a saucepan and bring it to a boil. While it is coming to a boil, stem the jalapeno pepper. If you like your Mexican food mild, remove the seeds. Chop the jalapeno finely. If you like things hot, retain the seeds when you chop the pepper. When the water comes to a boil, add the rice, garlic salt, and chopped jalapeno to the pan and return it to a boil. Turn the heat down to low and simmer it for 15 to 20 minutes or until the rice is tender. Check the rice after 15 minutes of cooking time and add more boiling water if necessary. While the rice mixture is cooking, chop the optional tomatoes and rinse the black beans by putting them in a strainer and running cool water over them. When the rice is cooked, stir the black beans into the rice mixture.

For non-vegetarian burritos, stir together the optional chicken and tomatoes or salsa.

Divide the bean mixture among the tortillas. Top with the optional tomato-chicken mixture and cheese. Roll the burritos up. Place them seam-side down on serving plates. Top them with cheese and microwave on low power or place the plates in a 300ºF oven until the cheese melts. Serve with other toppings of your choice. If you have more bean and chicken filling than you will use immediately, refrigerate or freeze it to use later. You can assemble the burritos using cold fillings and then warm them in the oven or microwave.

*Note: If you want to use less flexible tortillas, put each tortilla on a plate, top it with the fillings of your choice, and warm it in the microwave or oven.

Nutritional analysis per serving based on using 12 flour (wheat) tortillas: 185 cal, 12.3 g protein, 34.9
g carbohydrate, 3.2 g fat, 0.8 g sat fat, 18 mg cholesterol, 536 mg sodium, 4.9 g fiber
Serving size: 1 burrito
Servings per batch: 12
Diabetic exchanges per serving: 2 starch/bread + 1 very lean meat + ¼ veg + ¼ fat

Red Enchiladas

Ingredients:

1 green pepper, chopped

1 small to medium onion, chopped

2 teaspoons oil

1½ cups shredded chicken

8 ounces shredded Monterey jack cheese

1½ cups red chile sauce (½ batch, recipe on page 169) or canned enchilada sauce

12 corn tortillas, about 6 inches in diameter, or other "rollable" tortillas*

Cooking oil spray

In a frying pan, sauté the pepper and onion in the oil until they are soft. Add the chicken and cheese and about ½ of the enchilada sauce, or enough of the sauce to moisten the mixture.

Spread about ¼ to ⅓ cup of the sauce on the bottom of a 13 by 9 inch baking dish. Preheat your oven to 350°F.

Spray both sides of four tortillas with cooking oil spray. Stack them on a dish. Microwave them for 30 to 60 seconds or until they are warm and soft. Spoon $\frac{1}{12}$ of the chicken mixture down the middle of each tortilla, wrap each tortilla around the filling and lay it seam side down in the baking dish. Repeat with the remaining tortillas. Spread the remaining sauce over the enchiladas in the baking dish. Cover the dish with foil. Bake for 30 to 40 minutes or until they are heated through. Remove the foil and sprinkle the remaining cheese over the enchiladas. Bake for another 5 minutes or until the cheese is melted.

*Note: If the tortillas you want to use in this recipe crack when you try to roll them around the filling, assemble the ingredients for this recipe as an enchilada casserole (page 167).

Nutritional analysis per serving: 196 cal, 12.2 g protein, 19 g carbohydrate, 8.0 g fat, 3.9 g sat fat, 30 mg
cholesterol, 254 mg sodium, 2.3 g fiber
Serving size: 1 enchilada
Servings per batch: 12
Diabetic exchanges per serving: 1 starch/bread + ¾ very lean meat + ⅔ lean meat + ⅓ veg + 1 fat

Green Enchiladas

Ingredients:

8 to 12 ounces fat-free or low-fat sour cream
3 tablespoons skim milk
¼ teaspoon garlic salt or salt (optional)
3 cups shredded chicken
8 ounces Monterey jack cheese
Green chile sauce – 2 cups canned green enchilada sauce or 1 batch (about 2½ cups) chunky homemade green enchilada sauce (recipe on page 169)
12 corn tortillas, about 6 inches in diameter, or other "rollable" tortillas*
Cooking oil spray

In a bowl, stir together the 8 ounces of sour cream, milk, and optional salt. Stir this mixture into the chicken thoroughly. Cut the cheese into 12 strips or "fingers" about ½ inch thick and wide and 4 to 5 inches long. Preheat your oven to 350°F.

Spread enough green chile sauce in the bottom of a 13 by 9 inch baking dish to thinly cover the bottom of the dish. This will be about ¼ to ½ cup of smooth canned sauce or about ¾ cup of chunky homemade sauce.

Spray both sides of four tortillas with cooking oil spray. Stack them on a dish. Microwave them for 30 to 60 seconds or until they are warm and soft. Spoon $\frac{1}{12}$ of the chicken mixture into each tortilla. Top with a cheese strip and roll the tortilla around the filling. Lay the enchiladas seam side down in the baking dish. Repeat with the remaining tortillas and filling. Spread the remaining sauce over the enchiladas in the baking dish. Dot with the remaining 4 ounces of sour cream if desired. Cover the dish with foil. Bake for 35 to 45 minutes or until they are heated through.

*Note: If the tortillas you want to use in this recipe crack when you try to roll them around the filling, assemble the ingredients for this recipe as an enchilada casserole (page 167).

Nutritional analysis per serving: 242 cal, 18 g protein, 21 g carbohydrate, 9.2 g fat, 4.8 g sat fat, 49 mg cholesterol, 240 mg sodium, 2.2 g fiber
Serving size: 1 enchilada
Servings per batch: 12
Diabetic exchanges per serving: 1⅛ starch/bread + 1½ very lean meat + ⅓ lean meat + ¼ milk + 1 fat

Easy Ground Beef Enchiladas

Ingredients:
1 pound extra lean ground beef
¾ cup chopped green bell pepper (about ½ of a large pepper)
¾ cup chopped red bell pepper (about ½ of a large pepper)
½ cup chopped onion (optional)
½ to 1 teaspoon chipotle chile powder or to taste (See "Sources," page 211)
    OR ¼ to ½ of a 7-ounce can chipotle peppers (optional)*
½ of a 6-ounce can of tomato paste
3 to 3¼ cups bottled salsa, divided (or substitute Salsa Fresca, page 170)
2 to 3 cups shredded low-fat cheddar cheese
12 6-inch corn tortillas, or other "rollable" tortillas**
Cooking oil spray

Cook meat, peppers, and onion in a skillet over medium heat, stirring and breaking the meat up, until the meat is brown throughout and the vegetables are soft. Drain any fat. If you are using the chipotle peppers, cut them into small pieces. Add the chipotle* peppers or powder, 1 to 1¼ cups of the salsa (use the smaller amount with the canned chipotles), and the tomato paste to the meat mixture and simmer about 5 to 10 minutes longer. Stir in 1½ cups of the cheese. Spread ½ cup of the salsa on the bottom of a 13 by 9 inch baking dish. Preheat your oven to 400°F.

Spray both sides of four tortillas with cooking oil spray. Stack them on a dish. Microwave them for 30 to 60 seconds or until they are warm and soft. Spoon about ⅓ cup of the meat mixture into each tortilla and lay them seam side down in the baking dish. Repeat with the remaining tortillas. Spread the remaining salsa over the enchiladas in the baking dish. Cover the dish with foil. Bake for 20 to 30 minutes or until they are heated through. Remove the foil and sprinkle the remaining cheese over the enchiladas. Bake for another 5 minutes or until the cheese is melted.

*Notes: *Unless you like your Mexican food extremely hot, do not use both chipotles and hot salsa. Chipotles or 1 teaspoon chipotle powder work well with mild or medium salsa.
    **If the tortillas you want to use in this recipe crack when you try to roll them around the filling, assemble the ingredients for this recipe as an enchilada casserole (page 167).

Nutritional analysis per serving: 210 cal, 14.9 g protein, 26 g carbohydrate, 5.7 g fat, 2.3 g sat fat, 17 mg cholesterol, 699 mg sodium, 2.6 g fiber
Serving size: 1 enchilada
Servings per batch: 12
Diabetic exchanges per serving: 1½ starch/bread + ⅓ very lean meat + 1 lean meat + ⅓ veg + ¼ fat

Shredded Chicken Filling

Ingredients:

4 pounds chicken breasts (boneless skinless breasts are convenient, or purchase a
    slightly heavier package if they are not boneless and skinless)
½ teaspoon salt
Water

If you are using chicken breasts with skin remove the skin. Place the chicken breasts in a large pot. Add the salt and enough water to cover the breasts. Bring it to a boil over high heat. Then reduce the heat and simmer it for 1 to 1½ hours. Cool the breasts in the broth for moist chicken. (You may refrigerate the whole pan at this point for several hours or overnight if you wish. The broth may gel if refrigerated overnight). When the breasts are cool, remove them from the broth and break apart the meat with your fingers, discarding any gristle or bone. Makes about 12 to 13 cups of shredded chicken. Use as much as needed in the recipes in this chapter within two days or freeze the leftover chicken in 1 or 2 cup portions for future use.

Nutritional analysis per 1 cup of shredded chicken: 211 cal, 41 g protein, 0 g carbohydrate, 4.2 g fat,
    1.2 g sat fat, 108 mg cholesterol, 88 mg sodium, 0 g fiber
  1 cup portions per batch: 12 to 13
  Diabetic exchanges per 1 cup portion: 5¾ very lean meat

Shredded Beef Filling

Ingredients:

2 to 2½ pounds chuck or round steak or roast
1 tablespoon chili powder or to taste
¾ cup beef broth OR ¾ cup water plus ½ Knorr-Swiss™ beef bouillon cube

Cut the steak or roast into its natural sections and trim as much of the fat and bone as possible. Cut the meat into 2-inch cubes and put it in the crock pot. Sprinkle the roast with the chili powder and pour the broth over the meat. Cover and cook on high for 8 to 10 hours or until the liquid has nearly dried out. Watch it and stir it as it nears the end of the cooking time so it does not actually dry out (which may allow the meat to burn).

If you used a chuck roast or steak, remove the meat from the pot and allow it to cool until you can handle it or refrigerate it overnight. Remove bones or gristle and shred it.

If you used a round steak or roast which contains very little gristle and no bones, you will be able to just stir the meat to break it up. In this case, if the liquid has not almost completely evaporated at the end of the cooking time, remove the lid from the pot and allow it to cook a little longer until the liquid is almost gone. Then stir the meat and break it up as you stir it before removing it from the pot.

Use as much of the shredded meat as needed in the recipes in this chapter within two days after cooking it or freeze the meat in 1 or 2 cup portions for future use. This recipe may be doubled if you want plenty of meat to freeze. Makes about 4 cups of shredded meat.

Nutritional analysis per 1 cup of shredded beef: 377 cal, 50 g protein, 1 g carbohydrate, 6.0 g fat, 2.3 g
    sat fat, 116 mg cholesterol, 116 mg sodium, 0.2 g fiber
1 cup portions per batch: 4
Diabetic exchanges per 1 cup portion: 7 very lean meat + $2\frac{3}{4}$ fat

Enchilada Casserole

Ingredients:

Chose any enchilada recipe on pages 163 to 165. For the green enchiladas, substitute shredded Monterey jack cheese instead of cheese cut into strips. Prepare the meat or meat-vegetable mixture as directed in the recipe. Set aside about ½ cup of the cheese.

Preheat your oven to 350°F. Spread about ½ cup of the sauce used in the recipe on the bottom of a casserole dish. Top with a layer of about ⅓ of the tortillas called for in the recipe. (Depending on the size and shape of the baking dish, you may have to cut the tortillas to fit the dish). Top the tortillas with half of the meat mixture, half of the non-reserved cheese, and ⅓ of the salsa or sauce. Repeat with another layer of tortillas, meat, cheese, and sauce. Top with a final layer of tortillas and the remaining sauce. Cover the dish with foil and bake for 30 to 45 minutes or until it is heated through. Remove the foil, sprinkle it with the reserved cheese, and bake it for another 5 minutes or until the cheese is melted.

Nutritional analysis per serving: same as for the enchilada recipe used
    Serving size: $\frac{1}{12}$ of the casserole
    Servings per batch: 12
    Diabetic exchanges per serving: same as for the enchilada recipe used

Fajitas

Ingredients:

1 large red bell pepper
1 large green bell pepper
1 medium onion
1 to 2 jalapeno peppers, or to taste
2 teaspoons oil
¼ teaspoon garlic salt or salt
¼ teaspoon oregano
8 to 10 flour, whole wheat, white spelt, or whole spelt tortillas*
2 cups shredded beef filling (page 166)
8 ounces shredded low-fat cheddar cheese
8 to 10 flour tortillas
Optional toppings of your choice
     Salsa fresca (recipe on page 170) or bottled salsa
     Guacamole (recipe on page 171)
     Reduced fat sour cream

Cut the peppers into strips about 1 inch wide. Slice the strips into ½ inch pieces. Coarsely chop the onion. Stem and slice the jalapenos. If you like your Mexican food mild, remove and discard the seeds. If you like it hot, do not discard the seeds. Put the vegetables into a frying pan with the oil and sauté until soft. If the meat mixture was made previously, reheat it. Divide the meat, vegetables, and cheese into 8 to 10 portions. Spread them down the center of the tortillas, roll them up, and place them seam-side down on serving plates. Microwave or heat in a 350ºF oven until the cheese is melted. Serve with the toppings of your choice.

*Note: If you want to make this recipe with a different kind of tortilla which is less "rolla-ble," put a tortilla on a serving plate, add the toppings, and eat it with a fork and knife.

Nutritional analysis per serving based on using flour (wheat) tortillas: 214 cal, 16 g protein, 21.8 g carbohydrate, 6.7 g fat, 2.2 g sat fat, 27 mg cholesterol, 328 mg sodium, 2.0 g fiber
Serving size: 1 fajita
Servings per batch: 10
Diabetic exchanges per serving: $1\frac{1}{5}$ starch/bread + $\frac{3}{4}$ very lean meat + 1 lean meat + $\frac{2}{3}$ veg + $\frac{2}{3}$ fat

Easy Red Chile Sauce

Ingredients:

> 3 tablespoons all purpose or white spelt flour
> 3 tablespoons chili powder or to taste
> ½ teaspoon garlic salt or salt
> 2 cups water
> 1 8-ounce can tomato sauce

In a saucepan, stir together the flour, chili powder, and salt. Add the water and stir until smooth and lump-free. Add the tomato sauce. Bring the pan to a boil over medium heat, stirring frequently. When it boils, reduce the heat and simmer it, stirring occasionally, for a few minutes until it thickens. Makes about 3 cups of sauce.

Nutritional analysis per cup: 77 cal, 2.8 g protein, 4 g carbohydrate, 1.5 g fat, 0.3 g sat fat, 0 mg
cholesterol, 733 mg sodium, 4 g fiber
1 cup portions per batch: 3
Diabetic exchanges per 1 cup portion: ⅓ starch/bread + 2 veg

Green Chile Sauce

Ingredients:

> 2 to 3 tablespoons oil
> ½ cup onion, finely diced
> 2 cloves garlic, minced
> 2 tablespoons all purpose flour, white spelt flour, or any white refined starch
>   such as cornstarch or tapioca flour or starch
> 1 cup chicken broth
> About 1½ cups canned diced green chile peppers (2 7-ounce cans or half of a
>   27-ounce can)
> 1 large tomato, diced
> 1 tablespoon fresh cilantro, chopped (optional)

Put two tablespoons of oil in a saucepan with the onion and garlic. Cook over medium heat for 5 to 10 minutes or until the onion is tender. If you are using flour and the vegetables seem to have "absorbed" most of the oil, add the additional one tablespoon of oil to the pan. If you are using flour, stir it into the vegetable mixture and cook it over medium heat for 2 to 3 minutes. If you are using a starch, stir it into the cool chicken broth. Add the broth to the pan and cook the mixture until thickened, about three or four minutes. Stir in the peppers and tomato and cook over low heat for 20 minutes, stirring frequently. Stir in the cilantro. Makes about 2½ cups sauce, or enough for one batch of green enchiladas.

Nutritional analysis per cup: 168 cal, 2.5 g protein, 14.8 g carbohydrate, 11.8 g fat, 0.9 g sat fat, 0 mg cholesterol, 798 mg sodium, 2.4 g fiber
   1 cup portions per batch: 2½
   Diabetic exchanges per 1 cup portion: $\frac{1}{3}$ starch/bread + $1\frac{2}{3}$ veg + 2 fat

Salsa Fresca

Bottled salsa is a great a time-saver, but the vinegar in it can be a problem for those on a low-yeast diet. Here is a recipe for salsa made without vinegar. It is delicious made with truly ripe tomatoes and other fresh vegetables.

Ingredients:

> 8 to 10 small (Roma are good) or 4 large ripe tomatoes
> 2 to 4 Serrano or jalapeno chiles, or to taste
> 1 clove of garlic
> 3 to 6 scallions with about 3 inches of the green tops, or to taste
> ¼ cup cilantro leaves (optional)
> Juice of 1 large lime or 1½ small limes, about 3 to 4 tablespoons
> ¾ teaspoon salt

Use a very sharp knife to chop the tomatoes into ¼ inch dice. Put the tomatoes and their juice into a bowl. Cut the stems off the chiles but do not remove the seeds. Chop the chiles very fine. Peel and mince the garlic. Slice the bulb end of the scallions in half and then cut the bulb and tops crosswise into pieces less than ¼ inch wide. Finely chop the cilantro. Add all of the chopped vegetables to the bowl with the tomatoes. Stir in the lime juice and salt thoroughly. If there is not enough "juice" to come to the top of the chopped ingredients, add a little water and stir thoroughly. Refrigerate the salsa for a few hours before serving to allow the flavors to meld. Makes about 4 cups of salsa.

Nutritional analysis per cup: 43 cal, 1.7 g protein, 9.7 g carbohydrate, 0.6 g fat, 0 g sat fat, 0 mg cholesterol, 456 mg sodium, 2.2 g fiber
   1 cup portions per batch: 4
   Diabetic exchanges per 1 cup portion: $1\frac{3}{4}$ veg

Guacamole

Ingredients:

> 1 large or 2 small avocadoes
> 1 to 2 slices of onion, chopped
> 1 tablespoon lemon juice
> ¼ teaspoon salt or garlic salt
> 1 large or 2 small tomatoes, chopped

Peel and seed the avocado(es). Put the avocado flesh, onion, lemon juice, and salt in a measuring cup and puree with a hand blender or puree them in a blender or food processor. Stir in the chopped tomatoes. Makes about 1½ to 1¾ cups of guacamole.

Nutritional analysis per cup: 211 cal, 3 g protein, 14.5 g carbohydrate, 17.7 g fat, 2.8 g sat fat, 0 mg
      cholesterol, 153 mg sodium, 6.9 g fiber
  1 cup portions per batch: 1¾
  Diabetic exchanges per 1 cup portion: 1½ veg + 3½ fat

No Fat Tortilla Chips

These chips are a crunchy, fun addition to special diets. While they're most traditional or "normal" when made with corn tortillas, try using tortillas made using other flours as well. If you keep an open mind, you will enjoy these other types of chips.

Ingredients:

> Tortillas, any kind
> Water
> Salt (optional)

Preheat your oven to 500°F. Dip the tortillas in water for a few seconds and then hold them up by the edge for a few seconds to drain off the excess water. Salt them lightly if desired. Stack them and cut them into 6 or 8 wedges. Place them in a single layer on a large baking sheet. (If you are making many chips and they don't all fit, don't crowd them onto the baking sheet; save the ones that don't fit for the next round of baking). Bake them for 4 minutes. Remove the baking sheet from the oven and turn the chips over. Bake them for an additional 3 to 4 minutes, watching them carefully, until they are brown. Remove them from the oven and cool them completely. Store them in an airtight container.

Nutritional analysis per serving: same as for the tortillas used if unsalted
    Diabetic exchanges per serving: same as for the tortillas used

Very Low Fat Tortilla Chips

How much fat these chips contain depends on how you spray them with oil. While cooking oil spray is supposed to contain "a trace" of fat, if you spray the chips for a long time, they'll have more fat than if you spray them quickly. People with food allergies should use cooking oil rather than cooking oil spray to avoid problems with additional ingredients in the spray.

Ingredients:

> Tortillas, any kind
> Cooking oil spray or cooking oil
> Salt (optional)

Preheat your oven to 500 °F. Quickly spray both sides of the tortillas with cooking oil spray on both sides or brush both sides with oil. Salt them lightly if desired. Stack them and cut them into 6 or 8 wedges. Place them in a single layer on a large baking sheet. (If you are making many chips and they don't all fit, don't crowd them onto the baking sheet; save the ones that don't fit for the next round of baking). Bake them for 4 minutes. Remove the baking sheet from the oven and turn the chips over. Bake them for an additional 2 to 4 minutes, watching them carefully, until they are brown. Remove them from the oven and cool them completely. Store them in an airtight container.

Nutritional analysis per serving: essentially the same as for the tortillas used if unsalted
    Diabetic exchanges per serving: essentially the same as for the tortillas used

Tortilla Torte

Ingredients:

2 8-ounce packages neufatchel cheese at room temperature
2 teaspoons grated lemon zest (peel)
1 tablespoon lemon juice
½ cup Fruit Sweet™ or honey
2 teaspoons cinnamon
7 to 8 flour, whole wheat, white spelt, or whole spelt tortillas, about 8 inches
   in diameter
Cooking oil spray
Additional cinnamon
4 cups sliced strawberries or peaches (optional)

Preheat your oven to 400 °F. Grate the outer yellow part (zest) of the peel off a small lemon. Cut the lemon in half and squeeze 1 tablespoon of lemon juice. Beat together the neufatchel cheese, lemon zest, lemon juice, Fruit Sweet™ or honey and 2 teaspoons cinnamon. Place a tortilla in an ungreased round cake pan. Spread it with about one-sixth of the cheese mixture. Add another tortilla and layer of cheese to the pan. Repeat until all the cheese mixture is used up. Top the final layer of cheese mixture with a tortilla. Spray the top of the tortilla with cooking oil spray and sprinkle with cinnamon. Bake, uncovered, until it is bubbly around the edges and lightly browned on top, about 25 to 35 minutes. Refrigerate until it is cool or overnight. Cut into wedges and serve with fruit if desired. Makes 8 to 12 servings.

Nutritional analysis per serving: 224 cal, 6.6 g protein, 30 g carbohydrate, 8.7 g fat,4.7 g sat fat, 21 mg
   cholesterol, 249 mg sodium, 1.0 g fiber
Serving size: $1/12$ of the torte
Servings per batch: 12
Diabetic exchanges per serving: 1¼ starch/bread + $2/3$ other carbs + ½ very lean meat + 1¼ fat

Special Occasion Breads and Desserts

Mmmm! Imagine walking by a bakery and smelling sweet breads and rolls baking inside! Your house can smell just as good, and if you make your own sweet breads and rolls, you can have them without sugar or hydrogenated fat.

Several of the bread recipes in this chapter call for dried fruit. Plain dried fruit which can be purchased from a health food store is the best kind to use. Candied or glacé fruit can be used instead but they contain sugar and a variable amount of liquid. Try to drain the liquid thoroughly before you add them to your bread, and check the dough often during the kneading part of the cycle because you may need to add an additional 2 to 4 tablespoons of flour to maintain the right consistency of the dough with the candied or glacé fruit.

Enjoy the experience of making these breads, the wonderful smells and tastes, and the health advantages of homemade treats!

Cinnamon Raisin Bread

Ingredients:	1½ pound loaf	1 pound loaf
Water	1⅛ cups	¾ cup
Oil	1½ tablespoons	1 tablespoon
Liquid lecithin (or may use additional oil)	½ tablespoon	1 teaspoon
Date sugar	⅓ cup	¼ cup
Salt	1 teaspoon	¾ teaspoon
Cinnamon	1½ teaspoons	1 teaspoon
Bread flour	3 cups	2 cups
Active dry yeast	1¾ teaspoons	1¼ teaspoons
Raisins	½ cup	⅓ cup

Cycle: Raisin bread or basic yeast bread. Put all of the ingredients except the raisins into your machine and start the cycle. When the "beep" to add raisins sounds, or 5 to 8 minutes before the end of the last kneading time, add the raisins to the machine. When the bread is done, drizzle with any sweet roll glaze, pages 200 to 201, if desired.

Nutritional analysis per serving: 78 cal, 1.8 g protein, 15 g carbohydrate, 1.3 g fat, 0 g sat fat, 0 mg cholesterol, 84 mg sodium, 0.5 g fiber
Serving size: approximately 1.0 ounce
Servings per large loaf: 24, **per small loaf:** 16
Diabetic exchanges: 1 starch/bread per serving

Gluten-Free Cinnamon Raisin Bread

Ingredients:	1½ pound loaf	1 pound loaf
Water	¾ cup	½ cup
Oil	2 tablespoons	1½ tablespoons
Eggs	3 eggs OR ¾ cup	2 eggs OR ½ cup
OR egg substitute	egg substitute	egg substitute
Salt	1 teaspoon	¾ teaspoon
Vitamin C crystals	⅛ teaspoon	Scant ⅛ teaspoon
Guar gum	4 teaspoons	3 teaspoons
Cinnamon	1½ teaspoons	1 teaspoon
Brown rice flour	2 cups	1⅓ cups
Potato flour	⅓ cup	¼ cup
Tapioca flour	⅓ cup	¼ cup
Date sugar	⅓ cup	¼ cup
Active dry yeast	2¼ teaspoons	1½ teaspoons
Raisins	½ cup	⅓ cup

Cycle: Raisin bread or basic yeast bread. Put all of the ingredients except the raisins into your machine and start the cycle. When the "beep" to add raisins sounds, or 5 to 8 minutes before the end of the last kneading time, add the raisins to the machine. When the bread is done, drizzle with any sweet roll glaze, pages 200 to 201, if desired.

Nutritional analysis per serving if made with eggs: 79 cal, 2.2 g protein, 9 g carbohydrate, 2.1 g fat, 0.2 g sat fat, 41 mg cholesterol, 91 mg sodium, 0.9 g fiber
Nutritional analysis per serving if made with egg substitute: 79 cal, 2.2 g protein, 9 g carbohydrate, 2.4 g fat, 0 g sat fat, 0 mg cholesterol, 94 mg sodium, 0.9 g fiber
Serving size: approximately 1.1 ounce
Servings per large loaf: 25, **per small loaf:** 17
Diabetic exchanges: 1 starch/bread per serving

Wheat-Free Cinnamon Raisin Bread

Ingredients:	1½ pound loaf	1 pound loaf
Water	1¼ cups	¾ cup + 1 tablespoon
Oil	1½ tablespoons	1 tablespoon
Liquid lecithin (or may use additional oil)	½ tablespoon	1 teaspoon
Date sugar	⅓ cup	¼ cup
Salt	1 teaspoon	¾ teaspoon
Cinnamon	1½ teaspoons	1 teaspoon
White spelt flour	3¾ cups	2⅝ cups
Active dry yeast	2¼ teaspoons	1¼ teaspoons

Cycle: Raisin bread or basic yeast bread. Put all of the ingredients except the raisins into your machine and start the cycle. When the "beep" to add raisins sounds, or 5 to 8 minutes before the end of the last kneading time, add the raisins to the machine. When the bread is done, drizzle with any sweet roll glaze, pages 200 to 201, if desired.

Nutritional analysis per serving: 80 cal, 2.3 g protein, 15 g carbohydrate, 1.2 g fat, 0 g sat fat, 0 mg cholesterol, 72 mg sodium, 0.7 g fiber
Serving size: approximately 1.0 ounce
Servings per large loaf: 28, **per small loaf:** 19
Diabetic exchanges: 1 starch/bread per serving

Cranberry Orange Bread

Try this recipe for Thanksgiving!

Use the recipe for "Cinnamon Raisin Bread," page 174, "Wheat-Free Cinnamon Raisin Bread," page 176, or "Gluten-free Cinnamon Raisin Bread," page 175, except substitute an equal amount of dried cranberries (craisins) for the raisins. For the cinnamon, substitute 1 tablespoon grated orange peel in the 1½ pound loaf or 2 teaspoons grated orange peel in the 1 pound loaf. If desired, drizzle with "Orange Glaze," page 201.

Nutritional analysis per serving: Essentially the same as for the recipe used. From the 1½ pound loaf whole batch values for the recipe you used, subtract 42 cal, 1 g protein, 10 g carbohydrate, and 3 g fiber and divide by the number of servings.
Serving size and number of servings per loaf: Same as in the recipe used
Diabetic exchanges: 1 starch/bread per serving

Challah

Ingredients:	1, 1½, or 2 pound machine
Water	1 cup
Fruit Sweet™ or honey	¼ cup
Oil	1 tablespoon
Liquid lecithin (or may use additional oil)	½ tablespoon
Salt	1 teaspoon
Optional saffron	A small pinch
OR yellow food coloring	OR several drops
Bread flour	3¼ cups
Active dry yeast	2¼ teaspoons

1 slightly beaten egg white OR "Bread or Bun Wash," page 111
A very small pinch of saffron OR 1 to 2 drops of yellow food coloring (optional)
Sesame seeds, about 2 teaspoons

Cycle: Dough cycle, using the ingredients above the line. When the cycle is finished, remove the dough from the machine. Divide it into 4 parts and roll each into a 20-inch long rope. Lay them side by side on an oiled baking sheet. Braid them by starting with the rope on the right side; bring it over its immediate neighbor, under the next rope, and over the last rope. Repeat the process over and over, starting from the right, until the loaf is all braided. Brush with the egg white or glaze mixed with saffron or food coloring and sprinkle with the sesame seeds. Allow to rise until double, 30 to 40 minutes, and bake at 375°F for 25 to 30 minutes, or until brown.

Nutritional analysis per serving: 81 cal, 2.3 g protein, 15 g carbohydrate, 1.2 g fat, 0 g sat fat, 0 mg cholesterol, 101 mg sodium, 0.3 g fiber
Serving size: approximately 1.1 ounce
Servings per loaf: 20
Diabetic exchanges: 1 starch/bread per serving

Wheat-Free Challah

Ingredients: **1, 1½, or 2 pound machine**

Water	1 cup
Fruit Sweet™ or honey	¼ cup
Oil	1 tablespoon
Liquid lecithin (or may use additional oil)	½ tablespoon
Salt	1 teaspoon
Optional saffron	A small pinch
OR yellow food coloring	OR several drops
White spelt flour	3¾ cups
Active dry yeast	2¼ teaspoons

1 slightly beaten egg white OR "Bread or Bun Wash," page 111
A very small pinch of saffron OR 1 to 2 drops of yellow food coloring (optional)
Sesame seeds, about 2 teaspoons

Cycle: Dough cycle, using the ingredients above the line. When the cycle is finished, remove the dough from the machine. Divide it into 4 parts and roll each into a 20-inch long rope. Lay them side by side on an oiled baking sheet. Braid them by starting with the rope on the right side; bring it over its immediate neighbor, under the next rope, and over the last rope. Repeat the process over and over, starting from the right, until the loaf is all braided. Brush with the egg white or glaze mixed with saffron or food coloring and sprinkle with the sesame seeds. Allow to rise until double, 30 to 40 minutes, and bake at 375°F for 25 to 30 minutes, or until brown.

Nutritional analysis per serving: 82 cal, 2.7 g protein, 15 g carbohydrate, 1.2 g fat, 0 g sat fat, 0 mg cholesterol, 88 mg sodium, 0.5 g fiber
Serving size: approximately 1.0 ounce
Servings per loaf: 23
Diabetic exchanges: 1 starch/bread per serving

Sugarplum Bread

Ingredients:	1, 1½, or 2 pound machine
Water	¾ cup
Fruit Sweet™ or honey	¼ cup*
Oil	1½ tablespoons
Liquid lecithin (or may use additional oil)	½ tablespoon
Salt	½ teaspoon
Nutmeg	½ teaspoon
Bread flour	2½ cups
Active dry yeast	2¼ teaspoons
Raisins	½ cup
Dried fruit (small pieces of cherries, pineapple, or papaya) OR glacé or candied fruit* (cherries or pineapple)	½ cup

Cycle: Dough cycle, using the ingredients above the line. Add the raisins and fruit at the "beep" for adding raisins or 5 to 10 minutes before the last kneading finishes. After the cycle ends, remove the dough and shape it into a ball on an oiled baking sheet. Allow it to rise in a warm place until double, about 50 to 70 minutes. Bake at 350°F for 35 to 50 minutes, covering it with foil if it browns too quickly.

*Note: If you use glacé or candied fruit rather than dried fruit, reduce the amount of sweetener to 3 tablespoons. You will probably also have to add 2 to 4 tablespoons flour with the fruit to maintain the right consistency of the dough. The bread will not be sugar-free if glacé or candied fruit is used. Sugar-free chopped dry fruit is available at health food stores.

Nutritional analysis per serving: 79 cal, 1.7 g protein, 15 g carbohydrate, 1.5 g fat, 0 g sat fat, 0 mg cholesterol, 88 mg sodium, 1.1 g fiber
Serving size: approximately 1.1 ounce
Servings per loaf: 23
Diabetic exchanges: 1 starch/bread per serving

Wheat-Free Sugarplum Bread

Ingredients: **1, 1½, or 2 pound machine**

Water	¾ cup
Fruit Sweet™ or honey	¼ cup*
Oil	1½ tablespoons
Liquid lecithin (or may use additional oil)	½ tablespoon
Salt	½ teaspoon
Nutmeg	½ teaspoon
White spelt flour	3 cups
Active dry yeast	2¼ teaspoons

Raisins	½ cup
Dried fruit (small pieces of cherries,	½ cup

    pineapple, or papaya) OR glacé or candied fruit* (cherries or pineapple)

Cycle: Dough cycle, using the ingredients above the line. Add the raisins and fruit at the "beep" for adding raisins or 5 to 10 minutes before the last kneading finishes. After the cycle ends, remove the dough and shape it into a ball on an oiled baking sheet. Allow it to rise in a warm place until double, about 50 to 70 minutes. Bake at 350°F for 35 to 50 minutes, covering it with foil if it browns too quickly.

*Note: If you use glacé or candied fruit rather than dried fruit, reduce the amount of sweetener to 3 tablespoons. You will probably also have to add 2 to 4 tablespoons flour with the fruit to maintain the right consistency of the dough. The bread will not be sugar-free if glacé or candied fruit is used. Sugar-free chopped dry fruit is available at health food stores.

Nutritional analysis per serving: 79 cal, 2.1 g protein, 15 g carbohydrate, 1.3 g fat, 0 g sat fat, 0 mg
    cholesterol, 78 mg sodium, 0.9 g fiber
  Serving size: approximately 1.0 ounce
  Servings per loaf: 26
  Diabetic exchanges: 1 starch/bread per serving

Mexican Holiday Bread

Ingredients:	**1, 1½, or 2 pound machine**
Water	¾ cup
Fruit Sweet™ or honey	¼ cup*
Oil	1½ tablespoons
Liquid lecithin (or may use additional oil)	½ tablespoon
Salt	¾ teaspoon
Grated orange peel	1½ teaspoons (packed)
Bread flour	2½ cups
Active dry yeast	2¼ teaspoons

Dried sweet (Bing) cherries, ½ cup
    OR glacé or candied cherries,* cut in half
Any glaze, pages 200 to 201, and additional cherries (optional)

Cycle: Dough cycle, using the ingredients above the line. Add the cherries at the "beep" for adding raisins or 5 to 10 minutes before the last kneading finishes. After the cycle ends, remove the dough and shape it into a ring on an oiled baking sheet. Allow it to rise in a warm place until double, about 30 to 45 minutes. Bake at 375°F for 25 to 40 minutes, covering it with foil if it browns too quickly. Cool the loaf completely on a cooling rack and, if desired, drizzle it with glaze and top the loaf with additional cherries.

*Note: If you use glacé or candied fruit rather than dried fruit, reduce the amount of sweetener to 3 tablespoons. You will probably also have to add 2 to 4 tablespoons flour with the fruit to maintain the right consistency of the dough. The bread will not be sugar-free if glacé or candied fruit is used. Sugar-free chopped dry fruit is available at health food stores.

Nutritional analysis per serving: 79 cal, 1.9 g protein, 15 g carbohydrate, 1.5 g fat, 0 g sat fat, 0 mg
    cholesterol, 72 mg sodium, 0.6 g fiber
  Serving size: approximately 1.1 ounce
  Servings per loaf: 21
  Diabetic exchanges: 1 starch/bread per serving

Wheat-Free Mexican Holiday Bread

Ingredients: **1, 1½, or 2 pound machine**

Water	¾ cup
Fruit Sweet™ or honey	¼ cup*
Oil	1½ tablespoons
Liquid lecithin (or may use additional oil)	½ tablespoon
Salt	¾ teaspoon
Grated orange peel	1½ teaspoons (packed)
White spelt flour	3 cups
Active dry yeast	2¼ teaspoons

Dried sweet (Bing) cherries,   ½ cup
    OR glacé or candied cherries,* cut in half
Any glaze, pages 200 to 201, and additional cherries (optional)

Cycle: Dough cycle, using the ingredients above the line. Add the cherries at the "beep" for adding raisins or 5 to 10 minutes before the last kneading finishes. After the cycle ends, remove the dough and shape it into a ring on an oiled baking sheet. Allow it to rise in a warm place until double, about 30 to 45 minutes. Bake at 375°F for 25 to 40 minutes, covering it with foil if it browns too quickly. Cool the loaf completely on a cooling rack and, if desired, drizzle it with glaze and top the loaf with additional cherries.

*Note: If you use glacé or candied fruit rather than dried fruit, reduce the amount of sweetener to 3 tablespoons. You will probably also have to add 2 to 4 tablespoons flour with the fruit to maintain the right consistency of the dough. The bread will not be sugar-free if glacé or candied fruit is used. Sugar-free chopped dry fruit is available at health food stores.

Nutritional analysis per serving: 79 cal, 2.3 g protein, 15 g carbohydrate, 1.4 g fat, 0 g sat fat, 0 mg
        cholesterol, 63 mg sodium, 0.5 g fiber
    Serving size: approximately 1.0 ounce
    Servings per loaf: 24
    Diabetic exchanges: 1 starch/bread per serving

Pannetone

Ingredients:	1, 1½, or 2 pound machine
Water	⅞ cup
Fruit Sweet™ or honey	3 tablespoons
Oil	1½ tablespoons
Liquid lecithin (or may use additional oil)	½ tablespoon
Salt	¾ teaspoon
Grated lemon peel (zest)	¾ teaspoon
Yellow food coloring (optional)	3 to 4 drops
Bread flour	3 cups
Active dry yeast	2¼ teaspoons
Golden raisins	¼ cup
Currants or dark raisins	¼ cup
Chopped citron (optional, or more raisins)	3 tablespoons

Cycle: Dough cycle, using the ingredients above the line. Add the raisins, currants, and citron at the "beep" for adding raisins or 5 to 10 minutes before the last kneading finishes. After the cycle ends, remove the dough, knead it briefly on a lightly floured board, and shape it into a ball. Place it on an oiled baking sheet or in an oiled and wax paper-lined 7 to 8-inch round casserole dish or pannetone pan. Allow it to rise in a warm place until double, about 30 to 45 minutes. Bake at 375°F for 40 to 50 minutes. Remove it from the baking sheet or casserole dish immediately.

Nutritional analysis per serving: 80 cal, 1.8 g protein, 15 g carbohydrate, 1.3 g fat, 0 g sat fat, 0 mg cholesterol, 64 mg sodium, 0.4 g fiber
    Serving size: approximately 1.0 ounce
    Servings per loaf: 24
    Diabetic exchanges: 1 starch/bread per serving

Blueberry Lemon Bread

Use the recipe for "Cinnamon Raisin Bread," page 174, "Wheat-Free Cinnamon Raisin Bread," page 176, or "Gluten-free Cinnamon Raisin Bread," page 175, except substitute an equal amount of dried blueberries for the raisins. For the cinnamon, substitute 1 tablespoon grated lemon peel in the 1½ pound loaf or 2 teaspoons grated lemon peel in the 1 pound loaf. If desired, drizzle with "Lemon Glaze," page 201.

Nutritional analysis per serving: Essentially the same as for the recipe used.
   Serving size and number of servings per loaf: Same as in the recipe used
   Diabetic exchanges: 1 starch/bread per serving

Wheat-Free Pannetone

Ingredients:	**1, 1½, or 2 pound machine**
Water	⅞ cup
Fruit Sweet™ or honey	3 tablespoons
Oil	1½ tablespoons
Liquid lecithin (or may use additional oil)	½ tablespoon
Salt	¾ teaspoon
Grated lemon peel (zest)	¾ teaspoon
Yellow food coloring (optional)	3 to 4 drops
White spelt flour	3⅜ cups
Active dry yeast	2¼ teaspoons
Golden raisins	¼ cup
Currants or dark raisins	¼ cup
Chopped citron (optional – or may add additional raisins and currants instead)	3 tablespoons

Cycle: Dough cycle, using the ingredients above the line. Add the raisins, currants, and citron at the "beep" for adding raisins or 5 to 10 minutes before the last kneading finishes. After the cycle ends, remove the dough, knead it briefly on a lightly floured board, and shape it into a ball. Place it on an oiled baking sheet or in an oiled and wax paper-lined 7 to 8-inch round casserole dish or pannetone pan. Allow it to rise in a warm place until double, about 30 to 45 minutes. Bake at 375°F for 40 to 50 minutes. Remove it from the baking sheet or casserole dish immediately.

Nutritional analysis per serving: 79 cal, 2.1 g protein, 15 g carbohydrate, 1.3 g fat, 0 g sat fat, 0 mg cholesterol, 62 mg sodium, 0.6 g fiber
   Serving size: approximately 1.0 ounce
   Servings per loaf: 25
   Diabetic exchanges: 1 starch/bread per serving

Hawaiian Bread

Ingredients:	**1, 1½, or 2 pound machine**
Coconut milk	½ cup
Pineapple juice concentrate, thawed	¼ cup
Pureed or thoroughly mashed banana (about 1 medium banana)	½ cup
Oil	2 teaspoons
Liquid lecithin (or may use additional oil)	1 teaspoon
Salt	½ teaspoon
Bread flour	2⅔ cups
Active dry yeast	1¾ teaspoons
Dry diced pineapple	⅓ cup
Unsweetened coconut (optional)	¼ cup
"Pineapple Glaze," page 201 (optional)	

Cycle: Dough cycle, using the ingredients above the line. Add the pineapple and coconut at the "beep" for adding raisins or 5 to 10 minutes before the last kneading finishes. After the cycle ends, remove the dough, knead it briefly on a lightly floured board, and shape it into a ball. Place it in an oiled pie dish. Allow it to rise in a warm place until double, about 40 to 60 minutes. Bake at 375°F for 30 to 40 minutes. Cover it with foil for the last 20 minutes of baking to prevent excessive browning. Remove it from the pie dish immediately. Cool the loaf completely on a cooling rack and, if desired, drizzle it with the glaze.

Nutritional analysis per serving: 80 cal, 1.8 g protein, 14 g carbohydrate, 1.9 g fat, 1.1 g sat fat, 0 mg cholesterol, 44 mg sodium, 0.4 g fiber
Serving size: approximately 1.0 ounce
Servings per loaf: 25
Diabetic exchanges: 1 starch/bread per serving

Wheat-Free Hawaiian Bread

Ingredients: **1, 1½, or 2 pound machine**

Coconut milk	½ cup
Pineapple juice concentrate, thawed	¼ cup
Pureed or thoroughly mashed banana (about 1 medium banana)	½ cup
Oil	2 teaspoons
Liquid lecithin (or may use additional oil)	1 teaspoon
Salt	½ teaspoon
White spelt flour	3 cups
Active dry yeast	2 teaspoons
Dry diced pineapple	⅓ cup
Unsweetened coconut (optional)	¼ cup
"Pineapple Glaze," page 201 (optional)	

Cycle: Dough cycle, using the ingredients above the line. Add the pineapple and coconut at the "beep" for adding raisins or 5 to 10 minutes before the last kneading finishes. After the cycle ends, remove the dough, knead it briefly on a lightly floured board, and shape it into a ball. Place it in an oiled pie dish. Allow it to rise in a warm place until double, about 40 to 60 minutes. Bake at 375°F for 30 to 40 minutes. Cover it with foil for the last 20 minutes of baking to prevent excessive browning. Remove it from the pie dish immediately. Cool the loaf completely on a cooling rack and, if desired, drizzle it with the glaze.

Nutritional analysis per serving: 81 cal, 2.1 g protein, 14 g carbohydrate, 1.9 g fat, 1.0 g sat fat, 0 mg cholesterol, 41 mg sodium, 0.6 g fiber
Serving size: approximately 0.9 ounce
Servings per loaf: 27
Diabetic exchanges: 1 starch/bread per serving

Jam Crescents or Ring

Ingredients:

1 batch of any sweet roll dough, pages 197, 199, or 200
⅓ to ½ cup all-fruit (sugar-free) jam
⅓ cup chopped walnuts or other nuts
2 teaspoons cinnamon
Any sweet roll glaze, pages 200 to 201 (optional)

Cycle: Dough cycle, using dough ingredients only. When the cycle finishes, knead the dough briefly on a lightly floured board. Oil a baking sheet. To make two crescents, divide the dough in half and roll each out to a 8-inch by 8-inch square. Spread the squares with the jam and sprinkle with the nuts and cinnamon, leaving about ¾-inch of dough plain around the edges. Roll up jelly-roll fashion, crimp the outer edge to the roll, and squeeze the ends together. Lay the rolls on the baking sheet with the seam down and curve them into crescent shapes. Using a sharp knife, make 7 cuts from the outer edge of the crescent to within about 1½-inch of the inner edge. Turn the slices on their sides, all facing the same direction.

To make a ring, roll the dough out to a 12-inch by 12-inch square. Spread all but a 1-inch margin on one edge of the square with jam, and sprinkle it with the nuts and cinnamon. Roll the square up jelly-roll fashion, beginning with the edge opposite the edge without jam. Lay the roll seam side down on the baking sheet. Using a sharp knife, make 11 cuts (at 1-inch intervals) through one side of the roll to within about 1½-inch of the other side of the roll. Form the roll into a circle with the cut edge on the outside. Turn the slices on their sides, all facing the same direction.

Allow the crescents or ring to rise in a warm place until double, about 40 to 50 minutes. Bake at 375°F until nicely browned, about 18 to 25 minutes for the crescents and 20 to 30 minutes for the ring. Remove from the baking sheet immediately and drizzle with glaze if desired.

Nutritional analysis per serving: To the whole batch values for the dough recipe used, add 528 cal, 10 g protein, 72 g carbohydrate, 22 g fat, 1.5 g saturated fat, 12 mg sodium, and 4 g fiber. Divide by the number of servings you cut your crescents or ring into to get the per serving values.
Diabetic exchanges: To the whole batch values for the dough recipe used, add 4½ fruit and 5½ fat exchanges. Divide by the number of servings you cut your crescents or ring into to get the number of exchanges per serving.

Streusel Coffee Cake

Ingredients:

1 batch of any sweet roll dough, pages 197 to 200
1 teaspoon grated lemon or orange rind (optional)

¼ cup flour, the same kind as used in the dough recipe
⅓ cup date sugar
1 teaspoon cinnamon
1 to 2 tablespoons oil (use larger amount with rice flour)
2 tablespoons finely chopped walnuts or other nuts

Cycle: Dough cycle using the ingredients above the line. Add the lemon or orange rind to the bread machine pan with the salt. When the cycle finishes, spread the dough in a lightly oiled 9-inch by 9-inch baking pan. In a bowl, stir together the flour, sweetener, and cinnamon. With a pastry cutter, cut in the oil. Stir in the nuts. Sprinkle the topping over the dough. Allow it to rise in a warm place until double, 30 to 60 minutes, depending on the kind of dough used. Bake at 375°F for 25 to 40 minutes, or until the coffee cake is browned on the top and bottom.

Nutritional Analysis: To the whole batch values for the dough recipe you used, add 515 cal, 7 g protein, 73 g carbohydrate, 22 g fat, 0.5 g saturated fat, 2 mg sodium, and 5 g fiber. Divide by the number of servings to get the per serving values.
Diabetic exchanges per whole batch: To the whole batch values for the dough recipe used add 1 starch/bread + 5 fat + 3½ fruit exchanges. Divide by the number of servings to get the exchanges per serving.

Monkey Bread

Ingredients:

1 batch of any sweet roll dough, pages 197 to 200
Cooking oil spray or cooking oil
½ cup date sugar
2 teaspoons cinnamon

Cycle: Dough cycle, using the dough ingredients only. When the cycle finishes, knead the dough briefly on a lightly floured board. Oil a 10-inch tube pan or a 2 to 3-quart round casserole dish. Stir together the date sugar and cinnamon. Divide the dough into 45 to 50 1-inch balls. Spray each ball lightly with cooking oil spray or brush it with cooking oil. Then roll the balls in the cinnamon mixture. Place the balls in the prepared pan. Sprinkle any remaining cinnamon mixture over the top of the balls. Let the bread rise in a warm place until double, about 35 to 50 minutes. Bake at 375°F for 35 to 45 minutes, or until brown. Remove from the pan immediately.

Nutritional analysis per serving: To the whole batch values for the dough you use, add 256 calories, 63 g carbohydrate, and 32 mg sodium. Divide by the number of servings.
Diabetic exchanges: To the whole batch values for the dough recipe you used, add 4 fruit exchanges. Divide by the total number of servings to get the exchanges per serving.

Fruit Kuchen

Ingredients:

1 batch of any sweet roll dough, pages 197 to 200
4 to 5 cups fresh or frozen blueberries or peeled, sliced apples or peaches
½ cup flour, the same kind as used in the dough recipe
½ cup quick cooking oats, uncooked
½ cup date sugar
3 teaspoons cinnamon
2 tablespoons oil

Cycle: Dough cycle, using the dough recipe ingredients only. When the cycle finishes, spread the dough in a lightly oiled 9-inch by 13-inch pan. Arrange the fruit evenly over the dough. In a bowl, stir together the flour, oats, date sugar, and cinnamon. Sprinkle the mixture with the oil and mix it in with your fingers. Sprinkle the oat topping over the fruit. Allow the kuchen to rise in a warm place until double, 30 to 60 minutes, depending on the kind of dough used. Bake at 350°F for 40 to 50 minutes, or until browned on the top and bottom.

Nutritional analysis per serving: To the whole batch values for the dough you use, add 1218 calories, 18 g protein, 225 g carbohydrate, 31 g fat, 37 mg sodium, and 28 g fiber. Divide by the number of servings to get the per serving values.
Diabetic exchanges: To the whole batch values for the dough recipe you used, add 5 starch/bread +11 fruit + 4 fat exchanges. Divide by the number of servings to get the exchanges per serving.

Freeform Apple Pie

Dough ingredients (1, 1½ or 2 pound machine):

½ cup + 1 tablespoon water
2 tablespoons apple juice concentrate, thawed
1 tablespoon oil
½ teaspoon salt
2 cups bread flour
1⅛ teaspoons active dry yeast

Filling ingredients:

5 to 6 cups peeled, sliced apples
1 teaspoon cinnamon
½ cup date sugar
⅛ cup tapioca flour or cornstarch

Cycle: Dough cycle, using the dough ingredients. When the cycle is finished, roll the dough out on a floured surface to a 16-inch circle. Transfer the dough to an oiled baking sheet. Mix the filling ingredients and put them in the center of the dough. Bring the edges of the dough up around the fruit to form a 10-inch pie, leaving a 5-inch circle of fruit exposed in the middle. Pleat the dough on the top of the pie and pinch the pleats together. Allow to rise in a warm place for 25 to 30 minutes. Cover the exposed fruit with a small circle of aluminum foil. Bake at 350°F for 40 to 55 minutes, or until brown on the top and bottom.

Nutritional analysis per serving: 231 cal, 4 g protein, 49 g carbohydrate, 2.3 g fat, 0 g sat fat, 0 mg cholesterol, 97 mg sodium, 0.7 g fiber
Serving size: ⅛ pie
Servings per batch: 8
Diabetic exchanges: 1½ starch/bread + 2 fruit per serving

Wheat-Free Freeform Apple Pie

Dough ingredients (1, 1½ or 2 pound machine):

½ cup water
2 tablespoons apple juice concentrate, thawed
1 tablespoon oil
⅜ teaspoon salt
2 cups white spelt flour
1¼ teaspoons active dry yeast

Filling ingredients:

5 to 6 cups peeled, sliced apples
1 teaspoon cinnamon
½ cup date sugar
⅛ cup tapioca flour or cornstarch

Cycle: Dough cycle, using the dough ingredients. When the cycle is finished, roll the dough out on a floured surface to a 16-inch circle. Transfer the dough to an oiled baking sheet. Mix the filling ingredients and put them in the center of the dough. Bring the edges of the dough up around the fruit to form a 10-inch pie, leaving a 5-inch circle of fruit exposed in the middle. Pleat the dough on the top of the pie and pinch the pleats together. Allow to rise in a warm place for 25 to 30 minutes. Cover the exposed fruit with a small circle of aluminum foil. Bake at 350°F for 40 to 55 minutes, or until brown on the top and bottom.

Nutritional analysis per serving: 234 cal, 4.5 g protein, 50 g carbohydrate, 2.5 g fat, 0 g sat fat, 0 mg cholesterol, 97 mg sodium, 0.5 g fiber
Serving size: ⅛ pie
Servings per batch: 8
Diabetic exchanges: 1½ starch/bread + 2 fruit per serving

Open Faced Pie

Dough ingredients (1, 1½ or 2 pound machine):

⅜ cup water
1 tablespoon + 1 teaspoon apple juice concentrate, thawed
2 teaspoons oil
¼ teaspoon salt
1¼ cups bread flour
¾ teaspoon active dry yeast

Cycle: Dough cycle. When the cycle is finished, carefully remove the dough from the machine without deflating it too much. Do not knead it. Roll it out on a lightly floured surface to a 12-inch to 13-inch circle. Transfer it to an oiled 9-inch to 10-inch pie plate. Trim the edges and fill with one of the fillings on the following pages. If desired, re-roll the scraps of dough and cut into wedges or into small shapes with cookie cutters. Lay them on top of the filling. Allow the pie to rise in a warm place for 25 to 30 minutes. Bake in a preheated 350°F oven for 40 to 50 minutes, covering with foil after the first 25 minutes.

Nutritional analysis per serving, crust only, must be added to filling: 78 cal, 2.1 g protein, 14 g
     carbohydrate, 1.3 g fat, 0 g sat fat, 0 mg cholesterol, 64 mg sodium, 0.5 g fiber
Serving size: ⅛ pie
Servings per batch: 8
Diabetic exchanges: 1 starch/bread per serving

Wheat-Free Open Faced Pie

Dough ingredients (1, 1½ or 2 pound machine):

⅓ cup water
1 tablespoon + 1 teaspoon apple juice concentrate, thawed
2 teaspoons oil
¼ teaspoon salt
1⅓ cups white spelt flour
⅞ teaspoon active dry yeast

Cycle: Dough cycle. When the cycle is finished, carefully remove the dough from the machine without deflating it too much. Do not knead it. Roll it out on a lightly floured surface to a 12-inch to 13-inch circle. Transfer it to an oiled 9-inch to 10-inch pie plate. Trim the edges and fill with one of the fillings on the following pages. If desired, re-roll the scraps of dough and cut into wedges or into small shapes with cookie cutters. Lay them on top of the filling. Allow the pie to rise in a warm place for 25 to 30 minutes. Bake in a preheated 350°F oven for 40 to 50 minutes, covering with foil after the first 25 minutes.

Nutritional analysis per serving, crust only, must be added to filling: 85 cal, 2.8 g protein, 15 g
carbohydrate, 1.4 g fat, 0 g sat fat, 0 mg cholesterol, 64 mg sodium, 0.3 g fiber
Serving size: 1/8 pie
Servings per batch: 8
Diabetic exchanges: 1 starch/bread per serving

Apple Open Faced Pie Filling

Filling ingredients:

¾ cup apple juice concentrate, thawed
2 to 3 tablespoons quick cooking tapioca granules
5 to 6 cups peeled and sliced apples (about 6 to 7 apples)
1 teaspoon cinnamon

Prepare the filling while the dough cycle for the crust is running. Combine the apple juice and tapioca in a saucepan and allow them to stand for 5 minutes. Stir in the fruit. Bring the mixture to a boil and simmer for 10 to 15 minutes, or until the apples soften slightly. Allow the filling to cool for at least 30 minutes. Then put it into the pie crust prepared as on pages 192 or 193. Allow the pie to rise in a warm place for 25 to 30 minutes. Bake in a preheated 350°F oven for 40 to 50 minutes, covering with foil after the first 25 minutes.

Nutritional analysis per serving, filling only, must be added to crust: 110 cal, 0.3 g protein, 27 g
carbohydrate, 0.4 g fat, 0 g sat fat, 0 mg cholesterol, 7 mg sodium, 0.6 g fiber
Serving size: 1/8 pie
Servings per batch: 8
Diabetic exchanges: 2 fruit per serving

Blueberry Open Faced Pie Filling

Filling ingredients:

¾ cup apple juice concentrate, thawed
4 tablespoons quick cooking tapioca granules
24 oz. frozen unsweetened or fresh blueberries

Prepare the filling while the dough cycle for the crust is running. Combine the apple juice and tapioca in a saucepan and allow them to stand for 5 minutes. Stir in the fruit. Bring the mixture to a boil and simmer for 5 minutes. Allow it to cool for at least 30 minutes. Then put it into the pie crust prepared as on pages 192 or 193. Allow the pie to rise in a warm place for 25 to 30 minutes. Bake in a preheated 350°F oven for 40 to 50 minutes, covering with foil after the first 25 minutes.

Nutritional analysis per serving, filling only, must be added to crust: 104 cal, 0.4 g protein, 26 g carbohydrate, 0 g fat, 0 g sat fat, 0 mg cholesterol, 7 mg sodium, 4 g fiber
Serving size: $\frac{1}{8}$ pie
Servings per batch: 8
Diabetic exchanges: $1\frac{3}{4}$ fruit per serving

Cherry Open Faced Pie Filling

Filling ingredients:

1½ cups apple juice concentrate, thawed, or ¾ cup Fruit Sweet™
4 tablespoons quick cooking tapioca granules
2 16-ounce cans unsweetened (water-pack) tart pie cherries, drained

Prepare the filling while the dough cycle for the crust is running. If you are using the apple juice, boil it down to ¾ cup volume and allow it to cool slightly. Combine the tapioca and Fruit Sweet™ or cooled apple juice in the saucepan and allow it to stand for 5 minutes. Stir in the fruit. Bring the mixture to a boil and simmer for 5 minutes. Allow it to cool for at least 30 minutes. Then put it into the pie crust prepared as on pages 192 or 193. Allow the pie to rise in a warm place for 25 to 30 minutes. Bake in a preheated 350°F oven for 40 to 50 minutes, covering with foil after the first 25 minutes.

Nutritional analysis per serving, filling only, must be added to crust: 139 cal, 0.8 g protein, 35 g
carbohydrate, 0.1 g fat, 0 g sat fat, 0 mg cholesterol, 3 mg sodium, 0.9 g fiber
Serving size: ⅛ pie
Servings per batch: 8
Diabetic exchanges: 2¼ fruit per serving

Pumpkin Open Faced Pie Filling

Filling ingredients:

1 cup water
1 envelope of unflavored gelatin OR 1 tablespoon coarse agar flakes
OR 1½ teaspoons fine agar flakes
1 16-ounce can pumpkin
1 cup date sugar
1 teaspoon cinnamon
1 teaspoon nutmeg
¼ teaspoon ground cloves
¼ teaspoon allspice
¼ teaspoon ginger

Prepare the filling while the dough cycle for the pie crust is running. Put the water in a saucepan and sprinkle the gelatin or agar over the surface. Bring it to a boil and simmer until the gelatin or agar dissolves. Stir in the rest of the ingredients thoroughly. Put it into the pie crust prepared as on pages 192 or 193. Allow the pie to rise in a warm place for 25 to 30 minutes. Bake in a preheated 350°F oven for 40 to 50 minutes, covering with foil after the first 25 minutes. Chill thoroughly before serving.

Nutritional analysis per serving, filling only, must be added to crust: 94 cal, 1.1 g protein, 22 g
carbohydrate, 0 g fat, 0 g sat fat, 0 mg cholesterol, 6 mg sodium, 1.9 g fiber
Serving size: ⅛ pie
Servings per batch: 8
Diabetic exchanges: 1¼ fruit + 1 vegetable per serving

Peach Open Faced Pie Filling

Filling ingredients:

¾ cup apple juice concentrate, thawed
4 tablespoons quick cooking tapioca granules
5 cups peeled, pitted, and sliced fresh peaches OR 5 cups drained water-pack
    canned peaches OR 24 ounces frozen unsweetened peaches

Prepare the filling while the dough cycle for the crust is running. Combine the apple juice and tapioca in a saucepan and allow them to stand for 5 minutes. Stir in the fruit. Bring the mixture to a boil and simmer for 5 minutes. Allow it to cool for at least 30 minutes. Then put it into the pie crust prepared as on pages 192 or 193. Allow the pie to rise in a warm place for 25 to 30 minutes. Bake in a preheated 350°F oven for 40 to 50 minutes, covering with foil after the first 25 minutes.

Nutritional analysis per serving, filling only, must be added to crust: 112 cal, 0.8 g protein, 27 g
    carbohydrate, 0 g fat, 0 g sat fat, 0 mg cholesterol, 7 mg sodium, 2.5 g fiber
Serving size: ⅛ pie
Servings per batch: 8
Diabetic exchanges: 2 fruit per serving

Sweet Rolls and Doughnuts

Sweet Roll Dough

Ingredients: **1, 1½, or 2 pound machine**

Water	⅞ cup
Fruit Sweet™ or honey	⅓ cup
Oil	1½ tablespoons
Liquid lecithin (or may use additional oil)	1 tablespoon
Salt	¾ teaspoon
Bread flour	3⅛ cups
Active dry yeast	1¾ teaspoons

Cycle: Dough cycle

Nutritional analysis per batch of dough: 1726 cal, 43 g protein, 298 g carbohydrate, 36 g fat, 0 g sat fat, 0 mg cholesterol, 1514 mg sodium, 6 g fiber. (These values are for the dough only. Add the values for additional ingredients in the following recipes and divide by the number of servings to get the per serving values).
Diabetic exchanges for the whole batch: 22 starch/bread

White Spelt Sweet Roll Dough

Ingredients: **1, 1½, or 2 pound machine**

Water	⅔ cup
Fruit Sweet™ or honey	⅓ cup
Oil	1 tablespoon
Liquid lecithin (or may use additional oil)	1 tablespoon
Salt	¾ teaspoon
White spelt flour	3¼ cups
Active dry yeast	1¾ teaspoons

Cycle: Dough cycle

Nutritional analysis per batch of dough: 1765 cal, 54 g protein, 315 g carbohydrate, 34 g fat, 0 g sat fat,
    0 mg cholesterol, 1514 mg sodium, 19 g fiber. (These values are for the dough only. Add the val-
    ues for additional ingredients in the following recipes and divide by the number of servings to get
    the per serving values).
    Diabetic exchanges for the whole batch: 22 starch/bread

Gluten-Free Sweet Roll Dough

Ingredients:	**1, 1½, or 2 pound machine**
Water	½ cup
Fruit Sweet™ or honey	¼ cup
Oil	2 tablespoons
Eggs OR egg substitute	3 eggs OR ¾ cup egg substitute
Salt	1 teaspoon
Vitamin C crystals	⅛ teaspoon
Guar gum	4 teaspoons
Brown rice flour	2 cups
Potato flour	⅓ cup
Tapioca flour	⅓ cup
Active dry yeast	2¼ teaspoons

Cycle: Dough cycle. This dough can be used in Fruit Kuchen, page 189, Streusel Coffee
Cake, page 205, Cinnamon Rolls, page 226, or Monkey Bread, page 206.

Cycle: Dough cycle

Nutritional analysis per batch of dough made with eggs: 1900 cal, 54 g protein, 328 g carbohydrate, 52
    g fat, 5 g sat fat, 1029 mg cholesterol, 2269 mg sodium, 21 g fiber. (These values are for the
    dough only. Add the values for additional ingredients in the following recipes and divide by the
    number of servings to get the per serving values).
Nutritional analysis per batch of dough made with egg substitute: 1892 cal, 54 g protein, 328 g
    carbohydrate, 61 g fat, 0 g sat fat, 0 mg cholesterol, 2344 mg sodium, 21 g fiber. (These values
    are for the dough only. Add the values for additional ingredients in the following recipes and divide
    by the number of servings to get the per serving values).
    Diabetic exchanges for the whole batch: 24 starch/bread

Whole Wheat Sweet Roll Dough

Ingredients: **1, 1½, or 2 pound machine**

Water	1 cup
Fruit Sweet™ or honey	⅓ cup
Oil	1 tablespoon
Liquid lecithin (or may use additional oil)	1 tablespoon
Salt	½ teaspoon
Whole wheat flour	3 cups
Active dry yeast	2¼ teaspoons

Cycle: Dough cycle

Nutritional analysis per batch of dough: 1860 cal, 56 g protein, 326 g carbohydrate, 37 g fat, 0 g sat fat, 0 mg cholesterol, 1021 mg sodium, 14 g fiber. (These values are for the dough only. Add the values for additional ingredients in the following recipes and divide by the number of servings to get the per serving values).
Diabetic exchanges for the whole batch: 23 starch/bread

Whole Spelt Sweet Roll Dough

Ingredients: **1, 1½, or 2 pound machine**

Water	1 cup
Fruit Sweet™ or honey	⅓ cup
Oil	1 tablespoon
Liquid lecithin (or may use additional oil)	1 tablespoon
Salt	½ teaspoon
Whole spelt flour	3¾ cups
Active dry yeast	2¼ teaspoons

Cycle: Dough cycle

Nutritional analysis per batch of dough: 2032 cal, 63 g protein, 358 g carbohydrate, 38 g fat, 0 g sat fat, 0 mg cholesterol, 1017 mg sodium, 35 g fiber. (These values are for the dough only. Add the values for additional ingredients in the following recipes and divide by the number of servings to get the per serving values).
Diabetic exchanges for the whole batch: 25 starch/bread

Kamut Sweet Roll Dough

Ingredients: **1, 1½, or 2 pound machine**

Water	1⅛ cups
Fruit Sweet™ or honey	⅜ cup
Oil	1 tablespoon
Liquid lecithin (or may use additional oil)	1 tablespoon
Salt	½ teaspoon
Kamut flour	3¼ cups
Active dry yeast	2¼ teaspoons

Cycle: Dough cycle

Nutritional analysis per batch of dough: 2414 cal, 65 g protein, 471 g carbohydrate, 31 g fat, 0 g sat fat, 0 mg cholesterol, 1512 mg sodium, 77 g fiber. (These values are for the dough only. Add the values for additional ingredients in the following recipes and divide by the number of servings to get the per serving values).
Diabetic exchanges for the whole batch: 30 starch/bread

Sweet Roll Glaze

Ingredients:

½ cup powdered sugar
2 teaspoons water or milk
OR 1½ teaspoons water or milk plus ½ teaspoon vanilla

Mix ingredients together thoroughly and drizzle on sweet bread or rolls.

Nutritional analysis: To the whole batch values for the rolls or bread you use this glaze on add 240 calories and 60 g carbohydrate.
Diabetic exchanges: Not recommended for diabetics since this is almost pure sugar.

Lemon Sweet Roll Glaze

Ingredients:

½ cup powdered sugar
1 tablespoon lemon juice

Mix ingredients together thoroughly and drizzle on sweet bread or rolls.

Nutritional analysis: To the whole batch values for the rolls or bread you use this glaze on add 244 calories and 61 g carbohydrate.
Diabetic exchanges: Not recommended for diabetics since this is almost pure sugar.

Orange Sweet Roll Glaze

Ingredients:

½ cup powdered sugar
5 teaspoons orange juice concentrate, thawed

Mix ingredients together thoroughly and drizzle on sweet bread or rolls.

Nutritional analysis: To the whole batch values for the rolls or bread you use this glaze on add 288 calories, 1 g protein, and 71 g carbohydrate.
Diabetic exchanges: Not recommended for diabetics since this is almost pure sugar.

Pineapple Sweet Roll Glaze

Ingredients:

½ cup powdered sugar
2 tablespoons pineapple juice concentrate, thawed

Mix ingredients together thoroughly and drizzle on sweet bread or rolls.

Nutritional analysis: To the whole batch values for the rolls or bread you use this glaze on add 208 calories , 1 g protein, and 76 g carbohydrate.
Diabetic exchanges: Not recommended for diabetics since this is almost pure sugar.

Cinnamon Rolls

Ingredients:

1 batch of any sweet roll dough, pages 197 to 200
Cooking oil spray OR 2 teaspoons oil
½ cup date sugar (or if you must, substitute ¼ cup sugar)
2 teaspoons cinnamon
½ cup raisins
Any sweet roll glaze, pages 200 to 201 (optional)

Cycle: Dough cycle with the sweet roll dough ingredients. When the cycle is finished, remove the dough from the machine and use a lightly oiled rolling pin to roll it out to a 12-inch by 15 to 18-inch rectangle on a lightly oiled board. Spray the rectangle with cooking oil spray or brush it with oil. Sprinkle it with the sweetener, cinnamon, and raisins. Starting at the long side, roll the dough up jelly roll fashion. Cut the roll into 12 to 15 slices and put them cut side down in an oiled 13-inch by 9-inch pan. (Or for individual cinnamon rolls, cut the dough into 15 slices and put each slice cut side down into an oiled muffin cup). Allow them to rise in a warm place until double, about 35 to 50 minutes. Bake at 375°F for 20 to 30 minutes. Drizzle with sweet roll glaze if desired.

To make cinnamon rolls with gluten-free dough, when you remove the dough from the machine, pat it out into a 6-inch by 12-inch rectangle on a very well oiled board. Spray or brush it with oil. Sprinkle it with ¼ cup date sugar or ⅛ cup sugar, 1½ teaspoons cinnamon, and ¼ cup raisins. Roll it up carefully starting at the long edge and cut it into 9 slices. Put them in an oiled 8-inch or 9-inch square baking pan and allow to rise until double, about 30 minutes. Bake as above. The nutritional values to add to the values for the dough for gluten-free cinnamon rolls are half of those given below.

Nutritional analysis per serving: To the whole batch values for the dough recipe used add 611 calories, 2 g protein, 150 g carbohydrate, 57 mg sodium, and 6 g fiber. Divide the total by the number of servings made to get the per serving values.
Diabetic exchanges: To the whole batch values for the dough used add 10 fruit exchanges. Add to the exchanges per batch for the dough used and divide by the number of servings made to get the number of exchanges per serving.

Hot Cross Buns

Ingredients:

1 batch of any sweet roll dough, pages 197, 199, or 200
½ cup currants or dried blueberries
1 slightly beaten egg white or "Bread or Bun Wash," page 111
Any sweet roll glaze, pages 200 to 201, optional

Cycle: Dough cycle, using the dough ingredients only. Add the currants or raisins to the machine at the "beep" for adding raisins or 5 to 10 minutes before the end of the last kneading time. At the end of the cycle, remove the dough from the machine and knead it a few times on a lightly oiled board. Roll it to ½-inch thickness with a lightly oiled rolling pin. Cut rounds of dough with a 2½-inch biscuit cutter or glass. Place them on a baking sheet that has been sprayed with cooking oil spray or lightly oiled and allow them to rise in a warm place until double, about 40 minutes. Snip a shallow cross in the top of each bun with a very sharp scissors, knife, or lamé. Brush the tops of the rolls with the egg white or wash. Bake at 375°F for 15 minutes, or until lightly browned. If desired, use sweet roll glaze to pipe a cross into the cross cut on the top of each roll. Makes about 12 buns.

Nutritional analysis per serving: To the whole batch values for the dough recipe used add 220 calories, 3 g protein, 52 g carbohydrate, 5 mg sodium, and 1 g fiber. Divide the total by the number of buns made to get the per serving values.
Diabetic exchanges: To the whole batch values for the dough used add 4 fruit exchanges. Divide by the number of servings made to get the number of exchanges per serving.

Heart Healthy Danish

Ingredients:

1 batch of any sweet roll dough, pages 197, 199, or 200
2 teaspoons oil
⅓ cup + ¼ cup date sugar (may substitute sugar if you must)
2½ teaspoons cinnamon, divided
Cooking oil spray or cooking oil
½ cup chopped walnuts or other nuts
¼ cup all fruit (sugar-free) jam

Cycle: Dough cycle, using only the sweet roll dough ingredients. When the cycle is finished, remove the dough from the machine and divide it in half. On an oiled board, use a lightly oiled rolling pin to roll each half out to a 12-inch square. Brush each half with 1 teaspoon oil. Sprinkle each half with about ⅙ cup sweetener and ¾ teaspoon cinnamon. Roll the dough up jelly roll fashion. Cut the roll into 12 slices and put them cut side down at least 3 inches apart on an oiled baking sheet. Oil your hand and flatten the slices with your fingers to make them about 3 inches in diameter. (They may spring back some after you remove your hand). Allow them to rise in a warm place until double, about 30 to 40 minutes. Spray the tops of the rolls lightly with cooking oil spray or brush them with cooking oil and cover them with a piece of waxed or parchment paper. Use a rolling pin to flatten them to ¼-inch to ⅜-inch thickness. Mix together the remaining ¼ cup sweetener, 1 teaspoon cinnamon, and nuts. Sprinkle the rolls with the mixture. Cover them with the waxed or parchment paper and flatten them to ¼-inch to ⅜-inch thickness again. Let them rise until double again, about 30 to 40 minutes. Make an indentation in the center of each roll with your fingertip and fill it with ½ teaspoon jam. Bake at 375°F for 8 to 12 minutes. Drizzle with any sweet roll glaze, pages 200 to 201, if desired.

Nutritional analysis per serving: To the whole batch values for the dough recipe used add 824 calories, 12 g protein, 98 g carbohydrate, 37 mg sodium, and 11 g fiber. Divide the total by the number of Danish made to get the per serving values.
Diabetic exchanges: To the whole batch values for the dough used add 6 fruit exchanges + 1 lean meat exchange + 8 fat exchanges. Add to the exchanges per batch for the dough used and divide by the number of servings made to get the number of exchanges per serving.

Cinnamon Crisps

Ingredients:

> 1 batch of any sweet roll dough, pages 197, 199, or 200
> 2 teaspoons oil
> ⅓ cup + ¼ cup date sugar (may substitute sugar if you must)
> 2½ teaspoons cinnamon, divided
> Cooking oil spray or cooking oil
> ½ cup chopped walnuts or other nuts

Cycle: Dough cycle, using only the sweet roll dough ingredients. When the cycle is finished, remove the dough from the machine and divide it in half. On an oiled board, use a lightly oiled rolling pin to roll each half out to a 12-inch square. Brush each half with 1 teaspoon oil. Sprinkle each half with about ⅙ cup sweetener and ¾ teaspoon cinnamon. Roll the dough up jelly roll fashion. Cut the roll into 12 slices and put them cut side down at least 3 inches apart on an oiled baking sheet. Oil your hand and flatten the slices with your fingers to make them about 3-inch in diameter. (They may spring back some after you remove your hand). Allow them to rise in a warm place until double, about 30 minutes. Spray the tops of the rolls lightly with cooking oil spray or brush with cooking oil and cover them with a piece of waxed or parchment paper. Use a rolling pin to flatten them to ⅛-inch to ¼-inch thickness. Mix together the remaining ¼ cup sweetener, 1 teaspoon cinnamon, and nuts. Sprinkle the cinnamon crisps with the mixture. Cover them with the waxed or parchment paper and flatten them to ⅛-inch to ¼-inch thickness again. Immediately bake them at 400°F for 10 to 12 minutes.

Nutritional analysis per serving: To the whole batch values for the dough recipe used add 657 calories, 11 g protein, 56 g carbohydrate, 49 g fat, 22 mg sodium, and 11 g fiber. Divide the total by 24 to get the per serving values.
Diabetic exchanges: To the whole batch values for the dough used add 3.5 fruit + 1 lean meat + 8 fat exchanges. Divide by 24 to get the number of exchanges per serving.

Orange Rolls

Ingredients:

1 batch of any sweet roll dough, pages 197, 199, or 200
3 teaspoons oil
½ cup date sugar (may substitute ⅓ cup sugar if you must)
4 teaspoons grated orange peel, divided
"Orange Glaze," page 201 (optional)

Cycle: Dough cycle, adding 2 teaspoons grated orange peel to the machine with the salt. When the cycle is finished, remove the dough from the machine and divide it in half. Roll each half out to a 12-inch by 7-inch rectangle on a lightly oiled board. Brush each half with 1½ teaspoons oil. Sprinkle each half with ¼ cup date sugar and 1 teaspoon grated orange peel. Roll up jelly roll fashion starting with the long side. Cut each roll into 12 slices and place them cut side down on an oiled or nonstick baking sheet. Let rise until double, about 30 to 35 minutes. Bake at 375°F for 12 to 18 minutes. Cool and drizzle with "Orange Glaze," if desired.

Nutritional analysis per serving: To the whole batch values for the dough recipe used add 516 calories, 96 g carbohydrate, 13 g fat, and 48 mg sodium. Divide the total by 24 to get the per serving values.
Diabetic exchanges: To the whole batch values for the dough used add 3 fruit + 1 fat exchange. Divide by 24 to get the number of exchanges per serving.

Lemon Rolls

Make the same as "Orange Rolls," above, except substitute lemon peel for the orange peel and drizzle with "Lemon Glaze," page 201, if desired.

Nutritional Analysis: Same as for "Orange Rolls," above
Diabetic Exchanges: Same as for "Orange Rolls," above

Heart Healthy Doughnuts

Ingredients:

1 batch of any sweet roll dough, pages 197, 199, or 200
Cooking oil spray or cooking oil
1 batch of any doughnut topping or frosting, pages 207 to 208 (optional)

Cycle: Dough cycle. When the cycle is finished, roll the dough out to about ½-inch thickness on a lightly oiled board with an oiled rolling pin. Cut into doughnuts with a floured doughnut cutter. Lightly oil a baking sheet or spray it with cooking oil spray. Transfer the doughnuts to the sheet with a spatula and spray them lightly with cooking oil spray or brush them with oil. Let them rise in a warm place until double, about 30 to 40 minutes. Bake at 375°F for 10 to 15 minutes or until the doughnuts are just beginning to brown. Spray both the top and bottom of each doughnut lightly with cooking oil spray and immediately shake them in one of the toppings below. Or, if you wish to frost them, oil them while warm and then allow them to cool before frosting them with one of the frostings below.

Nutritional analysis per serving: Essentially the same as for the dough used. Divide the whole batch values for the dough used by the number of doughnuts made to get the values for each doughnut.
Diabetic exchanges: Divide the number of exchanges for a whole batch of the dough used by the number of doughnuts made to get the exchanges per serving.

Cinnamon "Sugar" Doughnut Topping

Ingredients:

¼ cup date sugar (or if you must, substitute sugar)
1 tsp cinnamon

Mix the sweetener and cinnamon in a plastic bag. Immediately after baking the doughnuts, spray each doughnut with cooking oil spray or brush it with cooking oil and shake the doughnuts one at a time in the bag with the cinnamon mixture while they are still warm.

Nutritional analysis per serving: To the whole batch values for the dough recipe used add 64 calories, 16 g carbohydrate and 2 g fiber. Divide the total by the number of doughnuts made to get the per serving values.
Diabetic exchanges: To the whole batch values for the dough used add 3 fruit exchanges. Divide by the number of doughnuts made to get the number of exchanges per serving.

"Powdered Sugar" Doughnut Topping

Ingredients:

¼ cup banana powder* OR powdered sugar

Put the banana powder or powdered sugar in a plastic bag. Immediately after baking the doughnuts, spray each doughnut with cooking oil spray or brush it with cooking oil and shake the doughnuts one at a time in the bag with the powder while they are still warm.

*Note: Banana powder, which is dehydrated ground bananas, can be purchased from The King Arthur Flour Baker's Catalogue. (See "Sources," page 211).

Nutritional analysis per serving: If you used the banana powder, to the whole batch values for the dough recipe used add 220 calories, 2 g protein, 53 g carbohydrate, and 2 mg sodium. For the powdered sugar, to the whole batch values for the dough recipe used add 120 calories and 30 g carbohydrate. Divide the total by the number of servings made to get the per serving values.
Diabetic exchanges: If you used the banana powder, to the whole batch values for the dough used add 4 fruit exchanges. Add to the exchanges per batch for the dough used and divide by the number of servings made to get the number of exchanges per serving. The powdered sugar is not recommended for use by diabetics

Vanilla Doughnut Frosting

Ingredients:

¾ cup powdered sugar
2 to 3 teaspoons water
½ teaspoon vanilla

Mix the sugar with the vanilla and enough water to make a thick frosting. Spread on the cooled doughnuts and sprinkle with nuts or coconut if desired.

Nutritional analysis per serving: To the whole batch values for the dough recipe used add 360 calories and 90 g carbohydrate. Divide the total by the number of doughnuts made to get the per serving values.
Diabetic exchanges: Not recommended for diabetics since this is almost pure sugar.

Chocolate Doughnut Frosting

Ingredients:

½ cup powdered sugar
2 tablespoons cocoa
2½ to 3½ teaspoons water

Mix the sugar and cocoa with enough water to make a thick frosting. Spread on the doughnuts and sprinkle with nuts or coconut if desired.

Nutritional analysis per serving: To the whole batch values for the dough recipe used add 274 calories, 2 g protein, 62 g carbohydrate, 2 g fat, and 1 mg sodium. Divide the total by the number of doughnuts made to get the per serving values.
Diabetic exchanges: Not recommended for diabetics since this is almost pure sugar.

References

American Diabetes Association/American Dietetic Association, *Family Cookbook,* Volumes I, II, and III. Prentice-Hall, Inc., Englewood Cliffs, NJ 07632, 1980, 1984, and 1987.

American Heart Association, *American Heart Association Cookbook*. Random House, Inc., New York, NY 10022, 1991.

Crook, William G., M.D., *Detecting Your Hidden Allergies*. Professional Books, 681 Skyline Drive, Jackson, TN 38301, 1988.

Crook, William G., M.D., *The Yeast Connection and the Woman*. Professional Books, Inc., Box 3246, Jackson, TN 38303, 1995.

Crook, William G., M.D. and Marjorie H. Jones, R.N., *The Yeast Connection Cookbook*. Professional Books, Inc., Box 3246, Jackson, TN 38303, 1989.

Dumke, Nicolette M., *Allergy Cooking with Ease,* Revised Edition. Adapt Books, Allergy Adapt, Inc., 1877 Polk Avenue, Louisville, CO 80027, 2007.

Dumke, Nicolette M., *Cooking 101: The Beginner's Guide to Healthy Cooking*. Adapt Books, Allergy Adapt, Inc., 1877 Polk Avenue, Louisville, CO 80027, 2002.

Dumke, Nicolette M., *Easy Breadmaking for Special Diets*. Adapt Books, Allergy Adapt, Inc., 1877 Polk Avenue, Louisville, CO 80027, 1995; Revised Edition, 2007.

Dumke, Nicolette M., *Easy Cooking for Special Diets: How to Cook for Weight Loss/Blood Sugar Control, Food Allergy, Heart Healthy, Diabetic and "Just Healthy" Diets – Even if You've Never Cooked Before*. Adapt Books, Allergy Adapt, Inc., 1877 Polk Avenue, Louisville, CO 80027, 2007.

Dumke, Nicolette M., *The Low Dose Immunotherapy Handbook: Recipes and Lifestyle Advice for Patients on LDA and EPD Treatment*. Adapt Books, Allergy Adapt, Inc., 1877 Polk Avenue, Louisville, CO 80027, 2003.

Dumke, Nicolette M., *The Ultimate Food Allergy Cookbook and Survival Guide: How to Cook with Ease for Food Allergies and Recover Good Health*. Adapt Books, Allergy Adapt, Inc., 1877 Polk Avenue, Louisville, CO 80027, 2007.

Fredericks, Carlton, Ph.D., *The New Low Blood Sugar and You*. Perigee Books, The Berkeley Publishing Group, 375 Hudson Street, New York, NY 10014, 1985.

Galland, Leo, M.D., *The Four Pillars of Healing*. Random House, New York, NY, 1997.

German, Donna Rathmell and Ed Wood, *Worldwide Sourdoughs from Your Bread Machine*. Bristol Publishing Enterprises, Inc., P.O. Box 1737, San Leandro, CA 94577, 1994.

Jones, Marjorie H., R.N., *The Allergy Self-Help Cookbook*. Rodale Press, Emmaus, PA 1984; Revised Edition, 2001.

Lai, Ada., *"The Magic Bread Letter"* Newsletter. The Magic Bread Letter, P.O. Box 337, Moss Beach, CA 94038.

Lewis, Sondra K. with Lonette Dietrich Blakely, *Allergy and Candida Cooking: Understanding and Implementing Plans for Healing*. Canary Connect Publications, 605 Holiday Road, Coralville, IA 52241-1016, 2006.

Rehberg, Linda and Lois Conway, *The Bread Machine Magic Book of Helpful Hints*. St. Martin's Press, New York, NY 10010, 1993.

Scala, James, *Eating Right For a Bad Gut*. Penguin Books USA, Inc., New York, NY 10014, 1990.

Starke, Rodman D., M.D. and Mary Winston, Ed.D., R.D., *American Heart Association Low-Salt Cookbook*. Random House, Inc., New York, NY 10022, 1990.

Sources of Special Foods and Products

BAKING POWDER, CORN-FREE:

Featherweight Baking Powder
The Hain Celestial Group, Inc.
4600 Sleepytime Drive
Boulder, CO 80301
(800) 434-4246
www.hain-celestial.com

BREAD INGREDIENTS, BAGS, KNIVES, ETC.;

Ingredients such as Instant Sourdough, Heidelberg Rye Sour, SAF™ and Red Star ™ yeast, etc.
The King Arthur Flour Baker's
    Catalogue
P.O. Box 876
Norwich, Vermont 05055
(800) 827-6836
www.kingarthurflour.com

BREAD MACHINES

Zojirushi BBCC-X20
The King Arthur Flour Baker's
    Catalogue
P.O. Box 876
Norwich, Vermont 05055
(800) 827-6836
www.kingarthurflour.com

CHIPOTLE CHILE POWDER:

Spices, Etc.
P.O. Box 2088
Savannah, GA 31402
(800) 827-6373
www.spicesetc.com

FLOUR:

MANY TYPES OF FLOUR –
UNBLEACHED, UNBROMATED
BREAD FLOUR, WHITE RYE, WHITE
WHOLE WHEAT, ETC.:

The King Arthur Flour Baker's
    Catalogue
P.O. Box 876
Norwich, Vermont 05055
(800) 827-6836
www.kingarthurflour.com

MANY TYPES OF FLOUR – RYE,
BUCKWHEAT, WHITE RICE, BROWN
RICE, KAMUT, ETC.

Arrowhead Mills
The Hain Celestial Group, Inc.
4600 Sleepytime Drive
Boulder, CO 80301
(800) 434-4246
www.hain-celestial.com

MANY TYPES OF FLOUR – POTATO FLOUR, TAPIOCA, ARROWROOT, TEFF, ETC.

Bob's Red Mill
Natural Foods, Inc.
5209 S.E. International Way
Milwaukie, OR 97222
(503) 654-3215
(800) 349-2173
www.bobsredmill.com

AMARANTH FLOUR:

Nu-World Amaranth, Inc.
P.O. Box 2202
Naperville, IL 60567
(630) 369-6819
www.nuworldfoods.com

MASA HARINA

The Quaker Oats Company
P.O. Box 049033
Chicago, IL 60604
(800) 694-7487
www.tortillamix.com
www.quakeroats.com

MILO AND MILLET FLOUR:

Purcell Mountain Farms
HCR 62 Box 284
Moyie Springs, ID 83845
866-440-2326
www.purcellmountainfarms.com

QUINOA FLOUR:

The Quinoa Corporation
Post Office Box 279
Gardena, CA. 90248
(310) 217-8125
www.quinoa.net

SPELT FLOUR (PURITY FOODS WHOLE AND WHITE SPELT):

Purity Foods, Inc.
2871 W. Jolly Road
Okemos, Michigan 48864
(517) 351-0231
www.purityfoods.com

GUAR GUM:

Bob's Red Mill
Natural Foods, Inc.
5209 S.E. International Way
Milwaukie, OR 97222
(503) 654-3215
(800) 349-2173
www.bobsredmill.com

SOURDOUGH CULTURES:

Sourdoughs International
P.O. Box 670
Cascade, ID 83611
(208) 382-4828
Fax: (208) 382-3129
www.sourdo.com

SWEETENERS

Fruit Sweet™, Grape Sweet™, Pear Sweet™

Wax Orchards, Inc.
22744 Wax Orchards Road S.W.
Vashon Island, WA 98070
(800) 634-6132
www.waxorchards.com

Date Sugar

NOW Natural Foods *(order through your health food store)*
395 S. Glen Ellyn Road
Bloomingdale, IL 60108
(800) 283-3500
www.nowfoods.com

TORTILLA MAKER, ELECTRIC:

VillaWare V5955 Grand Wrap Tortilla and Flatbread Maker

For a retailer, search this website:
www.villaware.com
Also available online from:
www.amazon.com and
www.pleasanthillgrain.com

TORTILLAS, SPELT OR WHOLE SPELT:

Rudi's Organic Bakery
3300 Walnut, Unit C
Boulder, CO 80301
(303) 447-0495
(877) 293-0876
www.rudisbakery.com

XANTHUM GUM

NOW Natural Foods *(order through your health food store)*
395 S. Glen Ellyn Road
Bloomingdale, IL 60108
(800) 283-3500
www.nowfoods.com

YEAST, regular and quick-rise, corn, gluten- and preservative-free:

Red Star Yeast and SAF Yeast
Universal Foods Corporation
Consumer Service Center
433 E. Michigan Street
Milwaukee, WI 53202
(414) 271-6755
www.redstaryeast.com

Red Star Yeast is a great information source but does not sell direct to consumers. To purchase Red Star™ or SAF™ yeast, contact:

The King Arthur Flour Baker's Catalogue
P.O. Box 876
Norwich, Vermont 05055
(800) 827-6836
www.kingarthurflour.com

Index of Gluten- and Wheat-Free Recipes by Grain Used

For gluten-free recipes, see the amaranth, garbanzo, quinoa, rice and teff sections below and three recipes in the corn section. All of the recipes in this index are wheat-free or (in the first section immediately below) can be made with grains other than wheat.

A VARIETY OF NON-WHEAT GRAINS CAN BE USED TO MAKE:

Appendix A: The Spelt-Wheat "Debate"

A great deal of confusion has risen concerning spelt recently. The United States Government is now requiring that foods be labeled to indicate whether they contain any of eight food allergens. As part of the implementation of this law, the FDA has declared that spelt is wheat. Although spelt and wheat are indeed closely related, they are two different species in the same genus. Spelt is *Triticum spelta* and wheat is *Triticum aestivum*. When asked why they had decided that spelt is wheat, an FDA official said that it was because spelt contains gluten. (They had no answer to the question of whether rye would also be considered wheat because it contains gluten, and indeed, bags of rye flour in the health food store are still labeled "wheat-free"). Spelt does indeed contain gluten and should not be eaten by anyone who is gluten-sensitive or has celiac disease, but the presence of gluten does not make spelt wheat.

The gluten in spelt behaves differently than the gluten in wheat in cooking. It is extremely difficult to make seitan from spelt. When making it from wheat, a process of soaking in hot water is used to remove the starch from the protein. If the same process is followed with spelt, the protein structure also dissolves in the hot water. Spelt seitan must be washed by hand very carefully under running cold water.

Because the gluten in spelt is more soluble than wheat gluten, making yeast bread with spelt is also different than making it with wheat. The individual gluten molecules join up more readily to form long chains and sheets that trap the gas produced by yeast. This means that it is possible to over-knead spelt bread. There are some bread machines that work quite well for wheat and even other allergy breads but are unacceptable for spelt bread because they knead so vigorously that they over-develop the gluten. See pages 32 to 33 for recommendations about bread machines to use for making spelt bread.

It is possible that the greater solubility of spelt protein makes it easier to digest than wheat. Undoubtedly, most people have had much less prior exposure to spelt than to wheat resulting in less opportunity to become allergic to spelt. Whatever the reason, there are many people who suffer allergic reactions after eating wheat but do not react to spelt. (I have talked to hundreds of them). Restricting one's diet unnecessarily, as the new law will undoubtedly lead people to do, is counterproductive to good nutrition. Consult your doctor about your own food allergy test results and follow the diet recommended for you, but do not unnecessarily restrict spelt consumption based on the faulty logic behind the new government labeling requirements.

Appendix B: Table of Measurements

When you make bread using a bread machine, measurements must be more precise than when you make it by hand. You will need to measure "unusual" amounts like ⅜ cup or ⅛ teaspoon. The easiest and most accurate way to do this is to have a liquid measuring cup with ⅛ cup markings, a set of dry measuring cups that contains a ⅛ cup measure, and a set of measuring spoons that has a ⅛ teaspoon. You can order such kitchen equipment from the King Arthur Flour Baker's Catalogue. (See "Sources," page 211). But while you are waiting to get those special measuring utensils, use this table to make your recipes work.

⅛ teaspoon	= ½ of your ¼ teaspoon measure	
⅜ teaspoon	= ¼ teaspoon + ⅛ teaspoon	
⅝ teaspoon	= ½ teaspoon + ⅛ teaspoon	
¾ teaspoon	= ½ teaspoon + ¼ teaspoon	
⅞ teaspoon	= ½ teaspoon + ¼ teaspoon + ⅛ teaspoon	
1 teaspoon	= ⅓ tablespoon	= ⅙ fluid ounce
1½ teaspoons	= ½ tablespoon	= ¼ fluid ounce
3 teaspoons	= 1 tablespoon	= ½ fluid ounce
½ tablespoon	= 1½ teaspoons	= ¼ fluid ounce
1 tablespoon	= 3 teaspoons	= ½ fluid ounce
2 tablespoons*	= ⅛ cup	= 1 fluid ounce
4 tablespoons	= ¼ cup	= 2 fluid ounces
5⅓ tablespoons	= ⅓ cup	= 2⅔ fluid ounces
8 tablespoons	= ½ cup	= 4 fluid ounces
16 tablespoons	= 1 cup	= 8 fluid ounces
⅛ cup	= 2 tablespoons*	= 1 fluid ounce
¼ cup	= 4 tablespoons	= 2 fluid ounces
⅜ cup	= ¼ cup + 2 tablespoons*	= 3 fluid ounces
⅝ cup	= ½ cup + 2 tablespoons*	= 5 fluid ounces
¾ cup	= ½ cup + ¼ cup	= 6 fluid ounces
⅞ cup	= ¾ cup + 2 tablespoons*	= 7 fluid ounces
	OR ½ cup + ¼ cup + 2 tablespoons*	
1 cup	= ½ pint	= 8 fluid ounces
1 pint	= 2 cups	= 16 fluid ounces
1 quart	= 4 cups OR 2 pints	= 32 fluid ounces
1 gallon	= 4 quarts	= 128 fluid ounces

*Note: In my experience, measuring tablespoons are all a little scanty of ¹⁄₁₆ cup, so 2 tablespoons is a little short of ⅛ cup. Therefore, if you need to measure, for example, ⅜ cup of liquid, it will probably be more accurate to "eyeball" an amount halfway between ¼ cup and ½ cup than to use ¼ cup plus two tablespoons.

General Index

Recipes appear in *italics;* informational sections appear in standard type.

Books to Help You with Your Special Diet

Easy Breadmaking for Special Diets contains over 200 recipes for allergy, heart healthy, low fat, low sodium, yeast-free, controlled carbohydrate, diabetic, celiac, and low calorie diets. It includes recipes for breads of all kinds, bread and tortilla based main dishes, and desserts. Use your bread machine, food processor, mixer, or electric tortilla maker to make the bread YOU need quickly and easily.

Revised Edition – ISBN 1-887624-11-2 or 978-1-887624-11-4 . . . . $19.95

Original Edition – ISBN 1-887624-02-3 . . . . $14.95

Easy Cooking for Special Diets: How to Cook for Weight Loss/Blood Sugar Control, Food Allergy, Heart Healthy, Diabetic and "Just Healthy" Diets – Even if You've Never Cooked Before. This book contains everything you need to know to stay on your diet plus 265 recipes complete with nutritional analyses and diabetic exchanges. It also includes basics such as how to grocery shop, equip your kitchen, handle food safely, time management, information on nutrition, and sources of special foods.

ISBN 1-887624-09-0 or 978-1-887624-09-1 . . . . $24.95

The Ultimate Food Allergy Cookbook and Survival Guide: How to Cook with Ease for Food Allergies and Recover Good Health gives you everything you need to survive and recover from food allergies. It contains medical information about the diagnosis of food allergies, health problems that can be caused by food allergies, and your options for treatment. The book includes a rotation diet that is free from common food allergens such as wheat, milk, eggs, corn, soy, yeast, beef, legumes, citrus fruits, potatoes, tomatoes, and more. Instructions are given on how to personalize the standard rotation diet to meet your individual needs and fit your food preferences. Contains 500 recipes that can be used with (or without) the diet. Extensive reference sections include a listing of commercially prepared foods for allergy diets and sources for special foods, services, and products.

ISBN 1-887624-08-2 or 978-1-887624-08-4 . . . . $24.95

Allergy Cooking With Ease **(Revised Edition)**. This classic all-purpose allergy cookbook was out of print and now is making a comeback in a revised edition. It includes all the old favorite recipes of the first edition plus many new recipes and new foods. Contains over 300 recipes for baked goods, main dishes, soups, salads, vegetables, ethnic dishes, desserts, and more. Informational sections of the book are also totally updated, including the extensive "Sources" section.

ISBN 1-887624-10-4 or 978-1-887624-10-7 . . . . $19.95

The Low Dose Immunotherapy Handbook: Recipes and Lifestyle Tips for Patients on LDA and EPD Treatment gives 80 recipes for patients on low dose immunotherapy treatment for their food allergies. It also includes organizational information to help you get ready for your shots.

ISBN: 1-887624-07-4 or 978-1-887624-07-7 . . . . $9.95

How to Cope With Food Allergies When You're Short on Time is a booklet of time saving tips and recipes to help you stick to your allergy diet with the least amount of time and effort.

$4.95 or FREE with the order of two other books on these pages

You can order these books on-line by going to www.food-allergy.org or by mail using the order form on the next page.

Mail your order form to:

Allergy Adapt, Inc.
1877 Polk Avenue
Louisville, CO 80027

Online orders can also be placed with Amazon.com at www.amazon.com.

Order Form

Ship to:

Name:

Street address:

City, State, ZIP code:

Phone number (for questions about order):

Item	Quantity	Price	Total
Easy Breadmaking for Special Diets* – Original Edition		$14.95	
Revised Edition		$19.95	
Easy Cooking for Special Diets*		$24.95	
The Ultimate Food Allergy Cookbook & Survival Guide*		$24.95	
Allergy Cooking with Ease*		$19.95	
The Low Dose Immunotherapy Handbook		$9.95	
How to Cope with Food Allergies When You're Short on Time		$4.95 or **FREE**	
Order any TWO of the first five books above and get *How to Cope* **FREE!**	Subtotal		
	Shipping – See chart below		
	Colorado residents add 4.1% sales tax		
	Total		

Shipping:
>   IF YOU ARE ORDERING JUST ONE BOOK, FOR SHIPPING ADD:
>> $4.00 for any one of the first four (starred*) books above.
>> $2.00 for either of the last two (non-starred) books above.
>   TO ORDER MORE THAN ONE BOOK, FOR SHIPPING ADD:
>> $6.00 for up to three starred* and two non-starred books
>> $9.00 for four starred* and up to two non-starred books

Call 303-666-8253 if you have questions about shipping calculations or large quantity orders.

Mail this order form and your check to the address on the previous page. Thanks for your order!

Printed in the United States
212487BV00003B/11/A